THE SECRETS OF STAYING YOUNG
(from the inside out)

**The latest information on how to become wrinkle resistant
and fight the signs of aging.**

by
Nina Anderson and Dr. Howard Peiper

Illustrated by
Richard Vail

**Revised edition:
OVER 50 LOOKING 30!**

Edited by Arlene Murdock

Published by SAFE GOODS
East Canaan, Connecticut

The Secrets of Staying Young
(from the inside out)

ISBN 1-884820-43-3
Library of Congress Catalog Card Number 98-61785
Revised edition
Over 50 Looking 30, The Secrets of Staying Young
Printed in the United States of America

Published by Safe Goods
283 East Canaan Rd.
East Canaan, CT. 06024
(860)-824-5301

PREFACE

The Secrets of Staying Young is the 1999 revised edition of the book, Over 50 Looking 30! The Secrets of Staying Young. Since we first wrote the book much new information has come across our desk. We wanted you to know the latest secrets for staying young, therefore we are offering you this completely revised edition. Besides expanding the chapter on Dis-eases, we would like you to be aware of the new secrets. We will highlight them here, but for details refer to their associated chapters.

Rhododendron caucasicum is a root herb that has been part of the daily intake for the people of the former Soviet Republic of Georgia. This natural substance has been used medicinally in foreign hospitals to treat heart disease, arthritis, gout, high cholesterol, blood pressure problems, depression, neuroses and psychoses and concentration problems. It is considered to be one of the keys to Georgian longevity. People in that country regularly live to be 120 years old and they even have a political party for the 100 plus age group. We have elaborated on this secret in the chapter *Herbs for Longevity*.

Two thousand years before written history began, a civilization known as the Sumerians learned how to harness the power of the sun. Their technology acknowledged that plants are a superior source of antioxidants and considered by some as the ultimate solar battery. They knew that complex chemical reactions convert fuel sources (the sun) to the primary energy compound, ATP. Harvested plants provide our cells with energized food so they can make this ATP, which is the only compound known to provide life force for all living things. The result is that our cells are nourished and now have the ability to slow the aging process as well as increase genetic efficiency. More on this process in the chapter *Greens and Live Foods*.

The benefits of growth hormone supplementation can be one or any of the following: improved stamina, sounder sleep, increase in energy, improved muscle tone, stronger nail growth, better digestion, weight loss, enhanced sexual function, increase in strength, improved mental processes, hair growth, less pain, reduction of wrinkles, diminished cellulite, eye sight improvements, emotional stability. This anti-aging supplement comes in many forms. We discuss the benefits of homeopathic remedies as being the safest way to augment your anti-aging regime with HGH. See the chapter on *Natural Treatments.*

Throughout the book we inserted new information on the benefits, of almonds, aloe, bioflavonoids, phytochemicals and co-factors. We also give possible causes for osteoporosis, cataracts, gout, age spots and hot flashes, as well as a frank discussion on the estrogen replacement therapy question. We hope you will find this revision comprehensive and enlightening.
-the Authors.

FOREWORD

A remark often made by middle-aged and older Americans, reflects a philosophical (if erroneous) concept that converts time from a dimension (duration) as a cause of sickness and bodily degeneration; "Well, of course I have a little arthritis; I'm growing older". In this philosophy, wrinkling of the skin, graying of the hair, cataracts and other degenerative diseases are seen as the inevitable and inescapable effects of time itself.

The authors of *The Secrets of Staying Young* present authoritative, accurate information concerning vital, complicated human nutritional processes in such an interesting and informative manner. Even as a physician, especially informed and interested in human nutrition, I learned much from this book.

Each chapter has such a personal impact and meaning for the reader, that they will stop and ponder as to how the facts and knowledge gained specifically apply to them. Many chapters will be reread several times. This book is well documented and is an excellent source of reference material. Here is a book for the physician and technically trained person as well as for the layperson. Non-medical people can expect technical knowledge expressed in direct yet simple understandable language, as far as food, diet and human nutrition are concerned. It will serve as a good review for even the physician, and will bring the nutritionist up to date.

How I wish I could have read this book before or during my medical school education, where today students tend to get lost among the trees of technical knowledge. It is difficult for them to grasp the broader perspectives; therefore, many doctors and their patients unfortunately suffer from malnutritional disease with resultant physical and mental deterioration.
-*James Balch, M.D.*

INTRODUCTION

Are you confused about the road to take for better health? Does your kitchen cabinet look like a vitamin factory and do you find that just when you settle into a new diet, you hear that science discovers that many of those foods actually harm you? Having been down that road for twenty-five years, we decided to research what the body really wants and pass this information along to you in a simple-to-read book. We take a good look at what happens inside our bodies that causes the aging process to rear its wrinkled head.

We always wondered if all the vitamins we popped into our mouths, really did anything in our bodies other than work our kidneys to excrete them. If all the nutritious foods we ate were really essential, then why did we still feel tired and get colds? Why were we starting to feel old and egads! we have reached middle-age and are facing mortality. This couldn't be! We can't get old! There must be a way to reverse time.

We found some interesting ways to slow the proverbial time clock down and keep us young-looking in the process. To our knowledge, no one has attempted to bring together in one book a good look at what causes aging and write it so the non-medical person can comprehend it. You have heard that there are sixty year-olds with thirty year-old minds and bodies. This proves that passing time does not mean you have to BE old. Much of it is a result of your mind set. To be old or to be young: the choice is yours.

In short, the calendar and clock, in themselves, are not toxic, nor are they the origin of degenerative changes and disease. It is important that this truth be grasped, otherwise there is little point in discussing the nutritional weapons that may halt, slow down or even reverse some of the symptoms and changes that we attribute to growing old. Before you load your body down with quantities of nutrients, based on information supported by manufacturers of those products or media advertising claims, let us help you understand a little about how the body works. We have attempted to do your homework for you and have weeded out many details, leaving the heart of the subject for you to comprehend. You can treat this material as an open door to walk through, absorb it and conduct further research using our extensive bibliography.

In treating the body as an eco-system within your skin this book gives information so you can stop polluting your personal planet, and start nourishing it. Our belief is that the mind controls our aging process. Not only can it convince you that you are young, but it can guide you to protecting your body from "terrorists" that can undermine it and cause sickness. We are not focusing on what already has been written such as vitamins, antioxidants, drugs, face lifts, etc. We simply provide you with a big picture so that you can plug in your pieces where they are necessary.

Anyone who speaks about longevity at some point will meet with resistance from people who adhere to the myths, or as we call them, excuses for not taking responsibility for their health. Just to impress upon you how shallow these myths are we present them in graphic form.

YOU HAVE TO DIE OF SOMETHING!

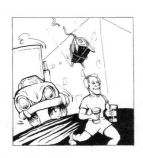

This is the most popular excuse people give for not taking care of their bodies. Smokers, drinkers, couch potatoes, sugarholics, vegetable haters, etc. All would rationalize that no matter what they did to themselves, they would eventually die. Ah, but what of the quality of life while living?

YOU ARE WHAT YOU EAT!

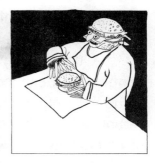

Obviously, eating burgers will not make you a burgerhead, but popular processed, cooked foods can definitely get a reaction from our body. Digestive aids, laxatives, sedatives, drugs, energy drinks are only some of the fixes for the trauma we inflict on our insides because of our eating habits, lifestyles and mental states. There is a link between our insides and outsides. The more we "trash" our insides, the worse we look and feel.

EVERYTHING IN MODERATION

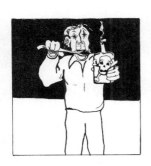

If this were true, we could take a wee bit of arsenic, lighter fluid and rat poison on a regular basis, with no harm. In the old days, before pesticides, pollution and processed foods, this may have been more true, but today these toxins accumulate in our bodies and accelerate the aging process and the onset of degenerative disease. Some things can be taken in moderation and even in abundance, but others should be avoided like the plague, and you should learn which are which.

THE MEDIA NEVER LIES!

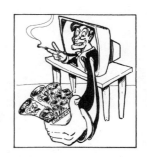

Advertising and media reporting can brainwash us into believing chemicals are good, drugs cannot harm, junk foods are healthy, and miracle cures are available for only $19.95. It is difficult for us to judge the truth. Remember when margarine was a heart saver? Now we find it contains evil trans-fats. It's a war out there, and you had better conduct your own research to determine what the real truth is, otherwise the yellow brick road will lead to the home for old crotchety geezers!

Our advisory staff has had success in treating and advising people for degenerative illness and the aging syndrome. We value their input and have asked them to contribute their professional expertise throughout these chapters. Manufacturers of products that support our research have included explanations of their products in our Resource Directory. Please educate yourself further by requesting supporting information from them. This book is printed in larger type for all of those people who have reached that magic age of needing reading glasses.

TABLE OF CONTENTS

THE BASICS OF LONGEVITY   13
FROM THE TABLE TO YOUR CELLS   17
WASTE REMOVAL   23
MINERALS   35
ENZYMES   45
ESSENTIAL FATTY ACIDS   55
GREENS AND LIVE FOODS   61
NATURAL TREATMENTS   71
PLANTS ASSURE LONGEVITY   79

     Garlic   80
     Rhodiola Rosea   84
     Rhododendron caucasicum   85

SKIN   89
HORMONAL IMBALANCES   93
DIS-EASES OF AGING   103

     Age spots   103
     Arthritis and osteoarthritis   104
     Baldness and thinning hair   107
     Blood clots   108
     Cancer   109
     Eye disorders   111
     Gout   114
     Heart disease   115
     Hot flashes   117
     Insomnia   118
     Memory   120
     Osteoporosis   122
     Panic attacks   126
     Parkinson's disease   126
     Prostate   130
     Sexual dysfunction   133
     Stress   135
     Varicose Veins   137

THINK YOUNG   139
FITNESS FOR YOUTH   147
APPENDIX   *(Nutritional supplement selection)*   157
RESOURCE DIRECTORY   159

THE BASICS OF LONGEVITY

The biggest secret in staying young is simple. In this chapter you will see how easy it is to maintain or regain your youth. To avoid the symptoms of aging, we need to create a partner with our body. We must give it the proper tools that build a strong immune system necessary to fight the aging process. These tools are minerals, enzymes and essential fatty acids. without which the body cannot function. The first secret revealed is to make sure you have these basics. We can best describe the basics necessary for health in an allegory that may be easy for you to remember.

THE BASICS.

MINERALS: YOUR BUILDING MATERIALS!

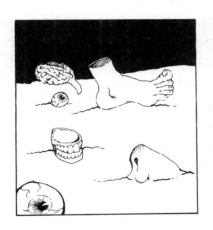

In order to build a healthy, youthful body, you must start with strong, efficient parts. Minerals, with electrolytes, are essential to the make-up of body parts and without these trace elements, the structure will not hold together very well. Over time, mineral deficiencies will cause the walls to groan, the siding will show cracks and blemishes, parts of the structure will sag and the roof might lose its shingles. Premature aging will be inevitable.

ENZYMES ARE THE CONSTRUCTION WORKERS!

Not much happens in the body without enzymes. Not only do they digest food, but they fight disease and regulate almost every function that supports life. Anytime you put cooked or processed food into your body, these construction workers must stop building the body, and run over to digest the food. Raw foods carry their own enzymes, so don't need to pull in the troops for help. When enzymes are diverted from their body building function, father time can do his dastardly deed of premature aging.

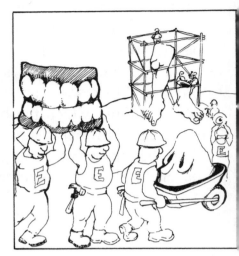

ESSENTIAL FATTY ACIDS ARE THE FOREMEN!

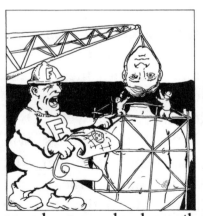

Construction workers must follow blueprints in order for the structure to go together properly. The foremen direct the operation and send messages that help get the job done properly. Without the essential fatty acids, the enzymes don't get proper messages. They may, in fact, do the wrong thing which contributes to the aging process. They must also be balanced, as one loud-mouthed foreman can do more to upset the harmony of the workers, than two complementary ones working for a common goal.

NUTRIENTS KEEP THE TERMITES AWAY!

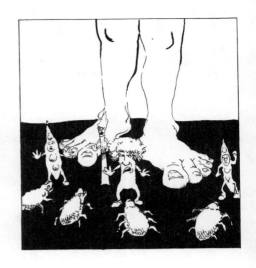

Disease, vermin, bugs, parasites, toxins can all whittle away at the body and cause its eventual demise. Fortifying the structure against these attackers is the key role of the immune system which itself must be fortified by nutrients we supply. Whole foods, micronutrients, kelp, wheatgrass, Chlorella, barley grass, veggies, chlorophyll and other antioxidants can keep the body's "dukes up" to defend itself against any toxic onslaught. Without these, we offer a happy home to chronic illness, senility and old, old skin.

FROM THE TABLE TO YOUR CELLS.

Maintaining a youthful body starts with what you eat. Since food is where we get most of our nutrients, it would make sense to address it in some detail. Food has to be digested (broken down into smaller particles), absorbed (taken from the intestines into the blood) and utilized (taken from the blood into the cells). Each of these steps is essential and if the elements ingested are missing any one of these steps, your body will not use these substances. Food is not a single entity such as oxygen or water. It consists of many different parts. These include carbohydrates (starches), protein (amino acids) and fats, the more forgotten vitamins, minerals, and most importantly, enzymes. Again, each of these substances is essential. Missing only one is the difference between life and death, between youth and aging.

For example, antioxidant supplementation would be futile if a person was deficient in the enzymes necessary to break down these antioxidants to a form which could fight the free-radicals (bad guys that contribute to aging). To make this easier to understand, let us tell you a story starting at your mouth and ending in your cells. Remember, your cells are where everything important happens. Metabolism, elimination of toxins, energy production and utilization of nutrients all occur in the blood. If any ingested substance doesn't get into the blood cell, it doesn't get used.

We normally assume that the digestive process starts with chewing. Actually, it begins as soon as you smell or even think of food. This starts your brain preparing digestive juices in anticipation of a meal. If you take *raw* food and put it in your mouth, chewing it breaks the cell membranes of the food, releasing enzymes that start digestion. Your saliva also releases the enzyme amylase, which starts digesting the starches in the food. If your meal is cooked, the enzymes in the food have been killed by the heating process. Although amylase helps with starch digestion, most of the food will have to wait until the pancreas secretes enzymes into the stomach. Chewing cooked food breaks the cells into smaller pieces, but since the enzymes in cooked food have been killed, no digestion takes place in the mouth. Food eaten raw does make less work for your body, in that most of the digestion is done by enzymes in the food.

If food is cooked above 118 degrees, enzymes are killed and your body has to do all the digestion by itself. On another note, if you don't chew your food, the enzymes found in your saliva will not be released, thus preventing starch digestion. It is very important to chew our food very well, much as a cow does. Next you swallow the food. It goes down into your stomach where the body secretes acids and enzymes to digest the proteins. The natural plant enzymes in raw food continue to digest the proteins, fats and the starches. Enzymes made by the saliva, stop working until the food gets into the small intestine, where there is less acid content than in the stomach. In the small intestine, enzymes are made by your body to digest the fats and starches. Again, if the food is raw, most of this work is done already. If it is cooked, your body has to put out a lot of energy to accomplish this task.

Breaking food down to a size appropriate for absorption is not an easy job. It is a lot of work for your body to digest food without the help of enzymes. This is why we often feel tired after eating a heavy meal. If you eat three meals a day, you may feel tired after each meal. One way to avoid this tired feeling is to replace the enzymes missing from cooked food by taking supplemental plant enzymes. We stress plant enzymes because they work throughout the entire digestive tract.

The small intestine is where absorption of the nutrients takes place. Nutrients are substances such as proteins, carbohydrates, fats, vitamins, minerals, and enzymes. In order for your body to use these substances, they must be broken down into their smallest components. Proteins are reduced to amino acids, fats into fatty acids, and carbohydrates into glucose. The food must also be sufficiently broken down to allow releasing of the vitamins and minerals. Food that is not broken down sufficiently suffers two fates.

The first, is that it may go through the intestines and feed the "bad" bacteria and yeast that invade your body. This encourages imbalance in the bowel and may facilitate the overgrowth of strains of bacteria and yeast. These strains damage the intestine and seep into the blood where the immune system has the task of getting rid of them. Secondly, the food may be absorbed in a partially broken down state. In the blood, products of this incompletely digested food are perceived by the immune system as a foreign invader, causing a negative immune system reaction which thinks the good food is really a bad invader. This can lead to fatigue or create allergies.

Let us not forget the part of food that cannot be digested. This is called fiber. For example when we examine grain, we find that the inner part is starch. This we break down into glucose and use for energy. The next outer part is the germ that contains all the vitamins, enzymes, and minerals we need in order to utilize the starch. If we eat the grain without the germ, we cannot use the starch and it will convert to fat as it builds up in the body. When the starch and the germ are both present we can utilize the most outer part of the grain to carry away the waste and reduce the fat build up. This is why whole grains are so important.

For example, stabilized rice bran is derived from the hull of rice (the brown part). When white rice is made, the brown layer is removed. This is the nutritionally beneficial part of rice and is a rich source of antioxidants (lipoic acid). Found in stabilized rice bran, lipoic acid has been measured to be 1,000 times more effective than vitamin E. Stabilized rice bran also contains compounds that dramatically reduce harmful cholesterol

19

levels (LDL), while increasing the good cholesterol (HDL), necessary for coronary health.

Elimination is the second most important process after digestion. For each particle of food the body uses, it produces an equivalent amount of waste. In order to eliminate this waste we need the fiber. This brings out the importance of eating foods that contain fiber. Eating whole foods is really all important, once you consider the nutrients and the fiber you are missing by eating processed grains or junk foods.

If we are successful in digesting our food, the nutrients are absorbed. As they circulate in the blood, they are absorbed and utilized by the cells. One requirement for nutrients to get to the cells, is proper blood circulation to the tissues. Blood is the very essence of life. It is the medium by which all of our organs obtain nutrients and facilitate waste elimination. Our brain, eyes, lungs, liver, kidneys, skin, hair, intestines, heart, blood vessels, and the rest of our body tissues, depend on this process for health.

It is often difficult to understand that whatever we find in the blood is found in every organ in the body. Whatever is not found in the blood is not usually found in our bodies. If the blood is clumped due to improper digestion, or circulation is poor due to lack of exercise, some cells may not receive enough nutrients. This can prevent waste elimination leading to those cells aging more quickly. It can also prevent oxygen from being transported to the tissues. Sometimes it is necessary for us to add an oxygen supplement to our diets, especially when we are engaged in strenuous exercise or are under stress. This not only helps the lungs do their job, but extra oxygen makes its way to the brain, enhancing our neuro-performance and assists in defeating a tell tale sign of aging, memory loss.

Consider whether or not the food you eat contains all the nutrients necessary for health. With the onset of present day chemical farming methods, much of our food is not only toxic, but the nutrient-depleted soil is deficient in vital substances that are needed to maintain a healthy body. Many of our foods such as corn, wheat, and some fruits are hybridized. What this means is that they have been weakened by genetic tampering. The reason for the tampering is to make the food look better and resist deterioration, not to improve its taste or nutritive content. No wonder that most Americans complain of being sick and low on energy.

To replace nutrients lost through poor quality foods, people often take high dosage supplements that may produce more symptoms than they help. A good example would be the process of taking ginseng to boost energy. Unfortunately, ginseng does not contain any fiber and if one's bowels are not functioning properly, the increased metabolism caused by the ginseng will serve to also increase the amount of waste produced by the body. It is important to always consider the whole picture, and the whole person in any therapy or supplement.

Another factor in the body's ability to utilize supplements is a term called bioavailability. This means that a substance is able to be used by the body. For instance, synthetic vitamin C alone is absorbed into the blood, but it is not easily utilized by the cells. If your body lacks the enzymes necessary to break down the vitamin pill, it will not be bioavailable. Because many people have poor digestion, they just may be creating very expensive toilet water.

Many of the supplements we take are simply eliminated as fast as we put them into our bodies. Nature designed nutrients to work together. If we isolate them from each other they lose their absorbability. Co-factors are substances that help other substances be assimilated. 100% pure vitamins do not work as well as 95% pure vitamins because the co-factors are missing. It is difficult for the layperson to know what should go with what, but you can always ask questions. Call the manufacturer and ask if their supplement contains all the co-factors needed for proper assimilation. If they don't know what you are talking about, choose another brand.

Even if we are diligent in our supplement selection, nutrients still may not be absorbed into the cell. This is due to the fact that most people today lack proper levels of trace minerals. Unfortunately, again due to modern farming methods, much of our food is mineral deficient. Levels in our water are waning as acid rain and topsoil runoff have sent the minerals scampering into the oceans. As we try to avoid water pollution, we filter our drinking water, which eliminates many of the minerals in the process. We definitely need to add back the minerals, as they are the building blocks for our whole physical structure.

WASTE REMOVAL

Key factors in promoting aging and degeneration are directly related to our lifestyles and habits. When we are born, our internal organs are absolutely clean and hopefully devoid of toxins. If we could preserve this pristine state, we would have baby soft skin throughout our lives and might delay degenerative disease. Unfortunately from the moment of birth, we are subjected to unfriendly bacteria, parasites and foreign toxins that all tax our immune system to the ultimate. If we could only think of our bodies as an eco-system in itself, we would be more diligent in avoiding pollution and maintaining that critical balance as nature intended.

Many of us take better care of our cars than of our bodies. We know that if we put water in our gas tank, our engine won't run. It's the same as if we put a poison in our body. But, if we only put a little water in the gas, our engine would still run, but not very well. This is what we are doing to our bodies with air and water pollution, toxic chemicals and our over-processed, additive laden foods. Since we cannot avoid many pollutants, and sometimes more than occasionally eat junk food, it is necessary to establish regular programs to remove this debris from our "personal planet."

To begin with, we must first understand the mechanics of our body. Our total digestive tract (from mouth to anus) is approximately 32 feet long. When we consume highly processed foods, this tubing becomes dangerously encrusted over the years. When our digestive system contains this intestinal barrier, it prevents nutrients from being absorbed into the blood stream. The body needs food, and if it is unable to access nutrients, the organs will receive less than perfect "fuel", and therefore not function properly.

The main anti-aging organs are the glands that produce hormones, and the organs which detoxify the body. Scientists believe that if hormones dwindle or lose their potency, the body will age. George Fahy of the Jerome Holland Laboratory of the American Red Cross in Rockville, Maryland, tells us that research shows if missing hormones are replaced, aging can be reversed. Since the glands that secrete these hormones are dependent on proper nutrition from the body, common sense would indicate that a starved gland would not work properly.

ENDOCRINE SYSTEM

PINEAL: Cone shaped gland at the base of the brain that secretes melatonin that helps synchronize biorhythms and is the "sleep" hormone.
PITUITARY: The body's "master gland" that stimulates the adrenals, thyroid, pigmentation-producing skin cells and gonads.
THYROID: Metabolism stimulating gland that controls body heat production and bone growth.
PARATHYROID: A gland that regulates the use and function of calcium and phosphorus in the body.
THYMUS: Located behind the breastbone, this gland is important in the development of cell-mediated immune responses.
ADRENALS: Crucial to controlling metabolism, this gland also produces hormones that maintain blood pressure and the body's salt and potassium balance.
PANCREAS: An abdominal organ that secretes insulin and glucagon to control the utilization of sugar, the body's energy source.
OVARIES: Female glands that produce estrogen and progesterone.
TESTES: Male glands that secrete testosterone to stimulate sperm production and development of male characteristics.

When glands do not work properly, they promote degenerative disease and a breakdown of the entire body's ecosystem. The body is also dependent on a proper acid/alkaline balance, know as pH. There is no ideal neutral state for acid/alkaline balance, as the intake of food and water constantly changes this balance. An acidic body fosters the condition for disease to get a foothold. This imbalance can be created by eating too many acid-forming foods and can also be caused by conditions of the body, such as vomiting, diarrhea, Diabetes or from some kidney diseases. It is extremely important when undertaking any detoxification program to monitor your pH and maintain a slightly alkaline condition (urine pH above 6.2). Some foods that promote alkalinity are vegetables, sprouts, potatoes, cereal grasses and most fruits. Sugars, meat, dairy, alcohol and most grains are acid.

As toxins are eliminated within our bodies, the eliminatory organs bear the responsibility of removing these foreign invaders. Flushing them out not only requires these organs to be in top physical condition, but it also demands lots of water. When man created alternatives to water (soda, coffee, alcohol), the conditions were right for creating constipation. Many liquids, especially those containing caffeine, are actually dehydrators and therefore it is absolutely necessary to drink at least eight glasses of water daily, or even more if you are removing poisons from your body.

Drinking water can be a risk in itself, as many sources are polluted, chlorinated, fluoridated and bacteria infested. Purified or bottled water is required for any detox program because we don't want to add more toxins during our cleansing program. Although our eliminatory organs can use lots of water to help them with their job, we also must be careful to replace lost electrolytes (minerals) that are a casualty of the flushing. If you have prepared your body properly by creating a slightly alkaline pH and consume a good bit of water on a regular basis, you can consider detoxing through different methods.

Blood cleansing can be initiated by going on a 3 to 7 day juice fast (organic). If you think you are really toxic, fast for only 3 days at one time because more aggressive programs may quickly release too many poisons creating an overload in the bloodstream. If you suspect you have heavy metal poisoning, beware of quick detox programs because you may find the rapid release of toxins many times causes you to become ill. As an alternative, aged garlic extract supplements can be added to your diet, because they assist in removing heavy metals.

Some herbs that can be used to detoxifiy the blood are red clover, hawthorn, alfalfa, nettles, sage, horsetail herb (silica), echinacea, licorice, garlic, milk thistle, pau d'arco, gotu kola, lemon grass and yerba santa. These herbs will also supply you with concentrated amounts of chlorophyll, helping to alkalize your pH. Detoxing may cause some symptoms such as headaches, nausea, bad breath, and body odor as the cleansing process progresses. Vitamin C is useful at this time to help keep the body alkaline, encourage oxygen uptake and promote creation of new tissue.

The liver, kidneys and the lymph glands are targets for disease, because as eliminatory organs they see their share of toxins and act as a storage bin for long periods of time. The liver is the body's most complex organ that converts everything we eat, breathe and absorb through the skin into life-sustaining substances. It is a highly condensed circulatory organ and produces natural antihistamines, manufactures bile to digest fats, excretes cholesterol, aids digestion and prevents constipation. It metabolizes proteins and carbohydrates, is a storehouse for vitamins and minerals and also secretes hormones and enzymes. We abuse it constantly, but it has the amazing ability to continue to function when 80% of its cells are damaged.

If you feel any of the following symptoms on a chronic basis, you may be in need of a liver cleanse: dizziness, dry mouth, slow elimination, mental confusion, unexplained weight gain, depression, major fatigue, PMS, constipation and food or chemical sensitivity. Since the skin is the body's largest organ, a liver cleanse might start there. Using an enzyme body wrap may also give great benefits to the skin. This can include alfalfa, ginger, dandelion root, spearmint, capsicum, cinnamon, and bladderwrack, in a base of lecithin, vegetable glycerin, aloe, olive oil, grapeseed oil and beeswax.

A liver flush tea could also be beneficial by taking 2-3 cups daily for one week. The tea could contain the herbs milk thistle seed extract, dandelion root, watercress, yellow dock root, pau d'arco, hyssop, parsley leaf, Oregon grape root, red sage, licorice, and hibiscus flower. As with all cleansing programs, you must maintain a slightly alkaline diet. As you rebuild the liver, you should avoid dairy, alcohol and caffeine. The addition of royal jelly, Chlorella and cereal grasses, and the anti-oxidants Vitamin A, C and E will help to restore the liver's strength. Raw liver extract (from clean sources) combined with aged garlic extract, vitamins B_1 and B_{12} become an excellent rebuilding tonic.

Detoxifying the liver and the blood cannot be accomplished effectively without also cleaning the digestive tract. If the body is constantly being poisoned from one source, the effects of a cleaner liver and blood will be short lived. People suffer from malnutrition and auto-intoxication because of a gradual build up of many layers of mucoid plaque substance in the intestinal tract. Just as hard water builds scale on the inside of your pipes, so do toxic eating habits affect the intestines.

When this plaque is present, there may be serious interference with the digestive process. Not only could constipation be a factor, but bigger than that, malnutrition. Any vitamins or healthful foods that we put in our bodies would be wasted money, as much of their nutritive elements would just be eliminated in the urine. Inside this encrusted wall lies the beginning of diverticulitis, colitis, colon cancer and a host of other diseases. The putrefied and stagnant pockets of poisons and harmful bacteria can fester and cause seepage into the bloodstream where these toxins travel to weaker parts of the body. This creates a breakdown of the immune system and can cause debilitating illness. Unfortunately symptoms resulting from toxic overload in the digestive tract are misdiagnosed, and the treatment may not be effective until the cause (toxic bowel) can be eliminated.

Something that no human ever wants to admit to is that they may have worms. Medical textbooks have revealed that over 55 million American children have worms, and the kids may come from clean environments. People are infected from flies, mites, food, pets, fingers, feces and from the air. Their ideal environment is the digestive tract, and they protect themselves from de-worming measures by hiding in the impacted layers of plaque. Over 134 kinds of parasites can live in the human body, with the World Health Organization naming parasitic diseases as among the six most harmful infective diseases in humans.

Parasites can cause many symptoms from digestive disturbances such as loss of sleep, headaches, anemia, coughing, blindness, skin ulcers and muscle pain, etc. Roundworms lay over 200,000 eggs per day and hookworms lay 5-10,000 eggs a day and can live for fourteen years. Once they are in your body, in addition to possible use of new drugs, a way to remove them is to clean your digestive tract and eliminate the parasites.

There are many ways to cleanse the colon including enemas and colonics (giant enemas that go "way up"). A more pleasurable way to foster this complete elimination of the digestive tract, is through herbal and oral ingestion method. Liquid bentonite and psyllium are key ingredients in moving plaque out of the system. Bentonite is a clay that acts like a sponge, absorbing toxic debris from the alimentary tract. It can absorb 180 times its own weight. It should be used with psyllium husk powder, which facilitates removal of the bentonite, along with the parasites and toxins. Obviously, lots of water should be taken with these substances to facilitate easy removal.

It is not uncommon for people to eliminate 20, 30 or 50 feet of mucoid plaque from their intestines with an outstanding effective digestive cleanse program such as that developed by Dr. Richard Anderson, N.D., N.M.D. Those who follow his program report that mucoid plaque is often eliminated in long pieces, resembling rubber or leather ropes, that may be easily saved in a colander for examination. Identifying what areas of the digestive tract are releasing plaque helps the cleanser to know what next steps they need to take in the cleansing process.

Along with these substances, the following herbs should be used for the reasons described:

Plantain breaks up intestinal mucoid substance. It is also good for the liver and kidney.

Barberry Bark is a powerful stomach and intestinal cleaner and blood purifier.

Myrrh helps build the immune system and helps rebuild the digestive system and remove gas.

Rhubarb Root act as a tonic to the liver and gall ducts. It helps cleanse the mucous membranes in the digestive system and is an excellent liver cleanser.

Fennel seed helps remove waste from all parts of the body, kills pinworms and calms the nervous system during the cleanse.

Ginger root removes some of the symptoms associated with the detoxifying process including headaches and an unsettled stomach. It also improves the effect of the other herbs used in the process.

Cascara Sagrada bark keeps things moving and rebuilds the peristaltic action in the intestines. It increases the secretions of the stomach, liver and pancreas thereby stimulating the removal of the mucoid substance.

Golden Seal stops infections and eliminates poisons.

Capsicum increases the effectiveness of the other herbs, and assists in the cleansing and rebuilding of the digestive system.

Red Raspberry Leaf helps prevent hemorrhages and diarrhea and creates an astringent and contracting activity within the intestinal membranes that helps dislodge mucoid crust.

Lobelia removes congestion and other obstructions from the body and helps with the elimination channels, especially the lymph.

herbal descriptions excerpted from Cleanse & Purify Thyself by Dr. Richard Anderson, N.D., N.M.D.

There are many other colon cleanse methods that use olive oil, lemon juice, apple juice, Epsom salts, etc. We hesitate advising you to use any of these treatments unless you are under the care of a naturopathic or allopathic physician. Because your body chemistry is finely tuned, any major change could have hazardous consequences. One of the side effects of detoxifying is emotional instability. When toxins are released, they may have memories attached to them that have been stored in the cells;

thus, emotions such as grief, anger and fear may be manifested. Be aware of this, and identify it as part of the cleansing process and not a mental problem. Detoxifying can also be assisted through homeopathic remedies. Removing toxins can normalize the function of the excretory system. Key remedies for this are Bryonia 10x, Nux vomica 10x and Chelidonium 10x.

Once you have detoxified, it is very important to rebuild the good bacteria in the intestinal tract, and to take foods and supplements that support the immune system. All this will benefit the anti-aging process. In the following chapters we cover nutritional aspects that support good health, and we suggest that you familiarize yourself with this material in order to make an educated decision about your own body. In the rest of this chapter, we will discuss the need for proper balance of intestinal flora.

The composition of friendly bacteria (probiotics) living in the intestines varies. There are over 100 trillion viable bacteria living together in symbiotic or antagonistic relationships inside the digestive system. They possess diverse enzymes that perform varied types of metabolism converting substances into compounds that can affect nutrition, physiologic function, drug efficacy, carcinogenesis, resistance to infection and aging. The intestinal flora can be upset (more bad guys than good guys) because of antibiotics, stress, influenza, excessive intake of alcohol and acid forming foods, exposure to disease and as part of the aging process.

When this upset occurs, our ability to process nutrients diminishes, we feel bloated, are constipated and develop a "leaky gut." Lack-luster eyes, poor skin, dull hair and excessive wrinkles are all subtle signs that friendly bacteria are missing from one's intestines. In a healthy, human being, Acidophilus bacteria exist from the upper part of the small intestine to the lower part of the small intestine and Bifidobacterium exist from the lower part of the small intestine to the large intestine. These lactic acid bacteria decrease the pH in the intestines (more acid), thereby producing substances that suppress harmful bacteria. They also activate macrophages (toxin eaters) which suppress the harmful bacteria. The large intestine is the main battle ground for the conflict against the bad bacteria.

In order for friendly bacteria to get to the large intestine, they must travel through stomach acids, which may kill them. When you take supplements of probiotics do so at the end of a meal, because they have a better chance of surviving stomach acid that has been diminished from food digestion. Important roles played by probiotics include the production of digestive enzymes, protecting the surfaces of intestinal mucous membranes, suppression of undesirable bacteria, reduction in gas and bad breath, production of many of the B vitamins and suppression of intestinal disorders. Lactobacillus also is undergoing research regarding its usage in cancer therapy.

There are many strains of probiotics. Most commercial yogurts contain only one, two or three. If the yogurt contains fruit or sugar, these bacteria will be killed. Plain yogurt with live cultures is best, but many supplements provide more concentrated quantities of probiotics. Kefir is an excellent source of live bacteria. Kefir is commonly made from a dairy source with added bacteria that has been allowed to ferment. When kefir is made from grain it becomes a complex, symbiotic mixture of microorganisms. This type of kefir is a staple of the people of the Republic of Georgia who are 36 times more likely to live to 100 years of age than Americans living in the United States. Grain kefir can have as many as 11 different species of probiotics and when freeze dried at low temperatures, can be added to a supplement. To help the probiotics do their job, homeopathic remedies can be used to normalize the function of the digestive system. For this purpose, Baptisia 10x and Lycopodium 15x can be taken fifteen minutes prior to meals.

In addition to taking probiotics, some cultivated herbal yeast supplements can help the body defend against the "bad guys." Nutritional yeast cells are rich in optimum combinations of many essential substances such as protein, carbohydrates, minerals, trace elements, amino acids, vitamins and enzymes. They can be extremely helpful in restoring strength to the beneficial bacteria.

In an interesting experiment conducted in 1977 by the Biochemical Laboratory of the Swiss College of Technology in Zurich, human cells (in vitro) were cultivated under hypo- and hyper-gravity conditions in the NASA space shuttle. Weightlessness in astronauts has been shown to inhibit the production of the lymphocytes necessary for the body's defense system. When a primary nutritional yeast supplement was introduced, the result showed that the activity of the cells, which is partially lost under microgravity, could be offset or compensated to a considerable extent. Other studies revealed that this substance has also been shown to have good infection fighting ability, especially in older animals. Nutritional yeast, derived from plants should not be confused with Brewer's yeast, a by-product of the brewing process.

If we relate back to the automobile analogy, we recognize the need to change our oil. If it has become clogged, it will affect our engine performance. Once the old contaminated oil (toxins) has been removed, we can add new oil (probiotics) and give our body a better chance to prevent illness and push back the effects of time.

A relatively new entry into the detoxification arena is ionized silver with electrolytes. Silver is considered to be one of the most universal antibiotic substances known. Because it is rare for a disease-causing organism to live in the presence of even minute traces of the chemical element silver, it is effective against more than 650 different pathogens. Silver does more than kill disease causing organisms. It also causes major growth stimulation of injured tissues and rapid healing from burns. It is effective in a detoxification program because it is rapidly fatal to parasites without any toxic effects on the human body. Virus, bacteria, fungus, yeast and mold are single cell organisms. Silver will kill the enzyme that allows them to live. As a result the microbe dies, and the white cells and larger tissue of the host remain unharmed.

Within the last few years, many silver products have appeared on the market. The best way to determine if a product is a true ionized (not colloidal) silver is to examine the ingredients. If the product contains a stabilizer or listed trace elements other than silver and electrolytes, the product may not be suitable. To be safe, the silver dosage recommended is 5 to 10 ppm or less. Electrolyte-based silver may be the icing on your colon cleansing cake.

Recommended reading:
•*Put Hemorrhoids and Constipation Behind You*, Kenneth Yasny, Ph.D.
  Safe Goods Publishing
•*The Body Ecology Diet*, Donna Gates with Linda Schatz
  BED Publications
•*Detoxification & Body Cleansing*, Linda Rector-Page, ND, Ph.D.
  Healthy Healing Publications
•*Cleanse & Purify Thyself, Book 1.5*, Dr. Richard Anderson
  Triumph Business
•*At Death's Door*, Dr. Richard Anderson,
  Triumph Business

MINERALS

If you want to live to be 100 and still have vitality and physical prowess, then this chapter is for you. Scientific research shows that the Hunza tribe, a 2000 year old civilization in the Himalayas, live far beyond the age of the average American. The Hunza quality of life far surpasses ours, as they experience little or no disease and age with increased mental alertness and sexual appetite. Today, it is not unusual for many of the people of the Republic of Georgia (part of the former Soviet Union), to live well beyond 100 in good health. In both cases the chief reason for longevity, is attributed to their mineral-rich drinking water. These glacial waters are abundant in the very minerals that are dangerously low in most commercial and public waters.

Both civilizations drink mineral rich water from mountain sources flowing underground and on the surface, down streams lined with rocks, which release not only calcium, but all other minerals and *trace-elements*. People advocating demineralized or purified water, like to emphasize that even if the minerals were useful, drinking water constitutes only a minor contribution to our daily intake of essential minerals and trace elements. They state that food sources contain all our mineral needs and there-fore, minerals from drinking water are insignificant, but they are dead wrong.

Obtaining minerals from vegetable sources is becoming more difficult each year, as the mineral content of our soils has decreased dramatically. Topsoil (the nutrient-rich ground cover) measurements have declined from 3 feet two hundred years ago, to less than 6 inches today. The decline is due partly to erosion, and largely to faulty agricultural techniques, such as over-grazing and the lack of crop rotation. Acid rain also contributes by lowering the pH of the soil, causing many of the remaining minerals to become locked up and therefore, unavailable to the plants. Needing sustenance, these plants substitute by taking up toxic pesticides, fertilizers and inorganic aluminum that entered the soil from the acid rain.

Food processing further depletes our food supply. Among the nutrients missing from and/or refined out of our food supply, are the vitally important trace minerals. These are needed in very small amounts by the body. They include such minerals as organic copper, zinc chromium, selenium, and iodine. In addition, certain macro minerals (those needed in large amounts) form the electrolytes, needed by the body to carry out all functions. Minerals play an integral role in the health of the immune system. For example, both the lack of zinc which is important in the production and health of our T-cells, and diminished levels of probiotics, lead to a weakening of the immune system. This causes increased vulnerability to opportunistic infections and yeast infections like Candida.

The maintenance and/or restoration of balance is the key. Basically we are healthy to the degree at which the body is able to maintain homeostasis, a steady state resulting from electrolyte balance. Electrolytes are minerals salts which are capable of conducting electricity when placed in a solution. In the body, the bloodstream provides the fluid medium, while the minerals are supplied from food and water, and in some instances nutritional supplements.

In the face of today's mineral deficiencies, the body's homeostatic capabilities have broken down. The resulting energy loss and imbalance have led to impairment of bodily functions and the development of disease. To restore homeostasis, the electrolyte minerals must be provided to the body in the proper form, combination and amount. The balance of minerals (mineral homeostasis) is as important a consideration in health, as their availability and assimilation. Minerals can compete with one another for absorption, especially if too much of one is available, and not enough of others. For example, too much zinc can unbalance copper and iron levels in the body and large amounts of calcium (2000 mg.) reduce absorption of magnesium, zinc, phosphorus and manganese.

A similar unbalancing of minerals can occur with excessive intake of single vitamins, either by producing a deficiency or increasing the retention of a particular mineral. A high intake of vitamin C decreases the absorption of copper and will contribute to a deficiency. Stress, aging, illness, athletic training and taking medicines all increase normal electrolyte requirements. Drugs may deplete minerals by increasing their excretion or interfering with mineral imbalance. Antibiotics will affect mineral absorption as well, and cause a decline in healthy intestinal bacteria. Antacids, laxatives, anti-convulsants, steroids, over consumption of protein and antibacterial agents are known to produce a deficiency of calcium and vitamin D. They exert a chelating action upon the calcium and antagonize the metabolic effects of vitamin D.

We are vibrating beings. The stronger the inner vibration, the healthier we are. The amplitude of body electricity is altered in exact proportion to the amount of alkaline and acid-forming chemicals internally present at any one moment. The pH determines whether a substance is alkaline or acid. The alkaline cells are tiny bundles of enzymes that produce energy and work within a very specific pH margin. The enzymes that work within the cell can only function when the fluid is as close to neutral pH as possible, except in the stomach, which is very acid. Anything that changes the pH of the cell environment can inactivate or change the level of activity of the cellular enzymes, possibly resulting in cellular starvation and cellular death.

A urine pH of 6.2 is best for human body function. However, it is impracticable for the average person to constantly check their urine throughout the work day. So, we have included a chart on the next page, that states what foods are acid forming and what foods are alkaline forming. By using the chart, you can even determine with a reasonable degree of certainty your alka-line-acid levels over an extended period of time.

With the average American diet very high in acid foods, we must protect the balances of the body's various systems with minerals. Since we are assaulting the body with high levels of acid foods, we must balance it with alkaline minerals. Since metabolic waste is in the form of some type of acid, the body often unites some of the base minerals with these waste acids and eliminates them through the urine. Very rarely is alkalinity a problem, although an overdose of the over-the-counter alkalizers has been known to produce this condition.

Acid/Alkaline Forming Foods
Fruits:
Acid: Cranberries, Strawberries, Sour fruits
Alkaline: Apples, Bananas, Citrus fruits, Grapes, Cherries, Peaches, Pears, Plums, Papaya, Pineapple, Berries, Apricots, Olives, Coconut, Dates
Vegetables:
Alkaline: All vegetables including potatoes, squash and parsnips
Grains:
Acid: Brown Rice, Barley, Wheat, Oats, Rye
Alkaline: Millet, Buckwheat, Corn, Sprouted grains
Meat/Dairy:
Acid: All meats and dairy products are acid except non-fat milk
Nuts/Seeds:
Acid: Cashews, Walnuts, Filberts, Peanuts, Pecans, Macadamia, Pumpkin, Sesame, Sunflower, Flax
Alkaline: Almonds, Brazil nuts, All sprouted seeds
Beans/Peas:
Acid: Lentils, Navy, Aduki, Kidney
Alkaline: Soybeans, Limas, Sprouted beans
Sugars:
Acid: All sugars except honey
Oils:
Acid: Nut oils, Butter, Cream
Alkaline: Olive, Soy, Sesame, Sunflower, Corn, Safflower, Canola, Margarine

In our opinion, acid wastes literally attack the joints, tis-sues, muscles, organs, and glands causing minor to major dysfunction. If they attack the joints, you might develop arthritis. If they attack the muscles, you could end up with myofibrosis (aching muscles). If they attack the organs and glands, a myriad of illnesses could occur. The more acidic we are, the lower our immune system becomes. The more protein (meat-based) we ingest, the more acidic our bodies become and therefore our immune system becomes weaker. Adding sugar to our systems enables the body to become even weaker.

Alkaline-forming substances create powerful and sustaining results that lead to superior health. The more extreme the deviations in pH, the more extreme the health symptoms one can experience. The goal in a day's time is to end up pH balanced but slightly more on the alkaline side than on the acid. There are products available that create alkaline water. This could be extremely beneficial when our diets are prone to be more acidic, but we must remember that our goal is to achieve homeostasis. To keep within a balanced pH range, a person using alkaline water should test their urine regularly to identify any overly alkaline condition the water could create.

We hear a lot today about benefits of "oxidative" therapies. These therapies utilize such substances as hydrogen peroxide and ozone which have the effect of increasing the amount of oxygen at the cellular level. Without adequate oxygen in our tissues, metabolism is adversely affected, as is the body's ability to eliminate toxins. Lack of oxygen in our bodies is reflective of a lack of oxygen in the body of the earth. As atmospheric carbon dioxide levels increase, oxygen levels in our environment decline, due largely to pollution and deforestation of our soils.

While the oxidative therapies are successful in terms of supplying the body with much needed oxygen, they supply that oxygen from the outside, doing nothing to improve the body's own oxidative ability. When vitamins, minerals and enzymes are supplied, we have the same situation. The body benefits as long as the substance is supplied, but nothing has been done to enable it to increase its own production of free radical scavengers. The key to enhancing the body's ability to produce enzymes is the

39

same key that normalizes all vital functions, and that is the restoration of homeostasis (electrolyte balance). Electrolytes are formed when certain minerals come together in solution and create electrical activity, providing energy for the body as water cascading down a rocky stream creates electrolytes.

Enzyme production in the body is dependent upon minerals which are the catalysts that make enzyme function possible. The key to oxygenating the body doesn't lie in providing extra oxygen from the outside. Restoring electrolyte balance is the answer. Electrolytes are nature's own oxygenators, and they provide the energy necessary for us to produce the anti-oxidant enzymes needed to destroy free-radicals, the by-products of oxidation. Electrolytes enhance tissue oxygenation, and aid in the reduction of free radical formation. The net result is that electrolytes can be a major factor in slowing down our skin's aging process.

Where do we find these electrolytes? Nature gives us water that flows and swirls over rocks, picking up the minerals and creating vortexes that produce an electrical charge. It also provides minerals absorbed from the ocean by sea vegetables. When choosing a mineral supplement, the form of the mineral is important. Large colloidal minerals have the least ability to be absorbed by the cell. The body takes the electrical charge from this mineral form and leaves the solid as residue. Unfortunately the body sometimes stores this debris in joints and kidneys causing illness. The next smallest form of mineral is chelated, which has a higher rate of absorption. It is quite often an extraction from plants, especially sea vegetables.

Further breaking down the mineral form, we find ionic, and when reduced further through a homeopathic process, we get a crystalloid. This is a substance, like a crystal, which forms a true solution and can pass through a living membrane. Crystalloid minerals contain electrolytes when they are electrically charged and found in solution. This form of mineral is assimilated 100 percent by the body. When nutritional supplements are taken with the crystalloid electrolytes, they become 100 percent bio-available (absorbed in the body where they are needed).

Serious age-related disorders like senility, are linked in several ways to electrolyte imbalance. Trace minerals are involved in the function of the minor blood vessels and capillaries in the brain, as well as the absorption of amino acids (protein), which the brain needs. The more efficient the circulation and transportation of oxygen, the better the memory remains intact over the years.

It is known that the brains of Alzheimer's patients contain abnormally high levels of aluminum. Aluminum has an enzyme inhibitory potential, and aluminum deposits prevent the brain from using vitamin B12. A lack of B12 allows the nerves to become hard. Some Alzheimer's patients also become very aggressive, which may give a further clue to an aluminum/Alzheimer condition. A study was done on aggressive boys in a detention home. Every one tested had abnormally high aluminum levels.

Sufficient intake of zinc, calcium and magnesium can stop aluminum from accumulating in the brain. Like plants, our bodies need a balance of minerals to prevent otherwise excessive levels of toxic minerals from being taken up by the cells and tissue. In recent studies, it was found that many mineral supplements contained inorganic aluminum. It would be prudent to query the manufacturer, and take only those that could insure you of being aluminum-free.

Mineral balance is critical, especially for the athlete. If copper is in short supply, iron utilization will decline and produce symptoms like fatigue and lack of stamina. In addition, the high volume oxygen intake during athletic exertion oxidizes blood cells faster than normal, and increases the chance of anemia. A high intake of meat and other proteins leads to an increase in the metabolic rate, part of which is achieved due to calcium and magnesium excretion. Loss of both these minerals can result in cramping, spasms, and irregular heart beat. Iron deficiency interferes with the formation of special enzymes in the body that affect muscle functions.

Zinc is another trace mineral that is lost during a workout, and could contribute to a male dysfunction. This mineral is used by the body for the production of a normal level of healthy sperm. In men who have a low sperm count, the replacement of lost electrolytes including zinc, brings their levels back to normal in a relatively short time (if there is nothing else causing the disorder). Impotence can also be associated with mineral deficiencies. It is thought that a significant number of men with this problem have atherosclerosis of the penile arteries, caused by a diet too high in certain fats, but most importantly, too low in trace minerals including chromium and manganese. Narrowed blood vessels restrict blood flow and limit erection. Chromium and manganese enable body systems to digest and excrete fats before they can become deposited on artery walls. Chromium also regulates mood swings, regulates blood sugar and blocks fat uptake.

Female athletes are especially prone to mild anemia or iron deficiency. Iron depletion is common and often goes undetected. Excessive physical activity often leads to loss of menstruation which stems from the body's depletion of minerals and its attempt to hang on to those which remain. Athletes may become deficient in many minerals, especially if the diet consists of refined foods, and if electrolytes are not replaced after workouts.

For any athlete or body builder, trace minerals or electrolytes need to be the first nutritional consideration. They work in the body to produce good assimilation and metabolism of nutrients, and the breakdown of proteins into amino acids. Minerals are involved in the building of new tissue, as well as keeping joints, bones, tendons and ligaments strong and flexible. They also help to keep the entire cardiovascular system healthy, quench damaging free radicals and maintain the strength of the cells and their fluid levels. Everything taken into the body needs trace minerals to make it work.

Minerals add back the life-force to water, but in addition, Tachyonization™ re-aligns water at a sub-molecular level, increasing the bio-energetic potential of the water. Using the accomplishments of scientists like Nikola Tesla and Henry Moray, the molecular structure of natural materials like silica, water, oil, cotton and silk can now be re-aligned, transforming them into antennae which attract life force energy. Drops of this water taken sublingually break the blood-brain barrier and instantly provide balancing life-force energy to the body, increasing the ability to focus and heightening the sense of well-being. Taken along with added minerals, you have one of the best secrets to longevity.

Recommended reading:
•*Crystalloid Electrolytes.*
Our body's energy source for the new millennium. Nina Anderson & Dr. Howard Peiper, Safe Goods Publishing
•*Electrolytes The Spark of Life*, Gillian Martlew, N.D. Nature's Publishing

ENZYMES

It has been suggested by many scientists that some people are old at 40 because of the lack of enzymes, while others are young at 80 because of the abundance of enzymes. As we age, if we don't add supplements, our body's enzyme supply decreases in number and activity level. Without a good supply of enzymes, antioxidants have a more difficult time of fighting wrinkles, a key sign of aging. Without enough enzymes, the body is unable to detoxify properly, reflecting this poisonous condition in our skin.

Stomach acid is essential for efficient nutrient absorption, and as people age, they lose the ability to secrete the necessary levels of hydrochloric acid required for proper digestion. At forty, people secrete only sixty-five percent of the normal levels of digestive enzymes, and at sixty-five it reduces to fifteen percent. Looking young depends on being young inside your body and adding an abundance of enzymes will head you in that direction.

Dr. Edward Howell, author and researcher of enzymes and nutrition for over fifty years, concludes that many, if not all degenerative diseases are caused by the excessive use of enzyme-deficient cooked and processed foods. He states, "the length of life is inversely proportional to the rate of exhaustion of the enzyme potential of an organism. The more the body's enzyme power must be used for digestion, the less there is for running the body."

Like money, enzymes are a form of power. They are active protein molecule catalysts, acting like microscopic hands performing practically all functions in the body. Vitamins and minerals have no function unless enzymes are present, because they are used by the enzymes to get the job done. Enzymes are present wherever chemical changes take place rapidly, without the added stimulus of heat. Since everything that takes place in physiology involves chemical change, enzymes must be present everywhere.

Your body cannot make vitamins and minerals, but it does have the power to make enzymes, which are energized protein molecules, the construction workers in the body that build the structure and keep it repaired. There are three primary groups of enzymes: *Metabolic enzymes* catalyze various chemical reactions within the cells, such as detoxification and energy production; *Digestive enzymes* are secreted along the gastrointestinal tract to break down food allowing nutrient absorption and include ptyalin, pepsin, trypsin, lipase, protease and amylase; Raw *plant enzymes* being protease, amylase, lipase and cellulase, are contained within the plant and used to digest that particular food.

Naturally-occurring enzymes in *raw* food are activated by the moisture and heat introduced during chewing. After this initial pre-digestion, the food moves to the upper stomach where it continues to break down, remaining in this location for an hour before gastric secretions move in. At this point, the enzymatic action is disabled by the acids and doesn't kick in again until the food reaches the small intestine, where pH is more alkaline. The presence of plant enzymes can be specific, as protease breaks down protein into amino acids, amylase breaks down carbohydrates into sugars, lipase breaks down fats into essential fatty acids and cellulase breaks down digestible fiber. Every raw food contains exactly the right amount and types of enzymes to digest that particular food. "An apple a day keeps the doctor away" works because of the nutrients supplied, but the enzymes provided in the fruit are actually only digesting the apple.

Certain enzymes need the proper pH range (acid/alkaline balance) to work. The pH range of the human gastrointestinal tract is approximately 1.5 to 8.0. Hydrochloric Acid (HCI) pH is 1.0, mixed with food it rises to 3.0. Its function is to maintain an acid pH so that the proteolytic enzyme pepsin, produced in the stomach, can work. Pancreatic (animal) enzymes work in a range of 7.8 to 8.3 and only provide digestive activity when the small intestine reaches 7.8. This is not often attained, due to inadequate secretion of bicarbonate. Concentrated plant enzymes work in a very broad range of 3.0 to 9.0, and therefore are the most effective type for supplementation.

Because our diets today consist mainly of cooked and processed foods, the body may have to supply enzymes for digestion. Storing foods at cold temperature make enzymes hibernate, only to be woken up once they are warmed. The optimal temperature for enzyme activation is 92-104°F, whereas cooking (above 118°) destroys enzymes. If the cooked food has no enzymes, the body must produce its own in order to digest the food. This also applies to foods that have been canned or processed (which is almost all commercially produced foods). If you just take inventory of what you eat in a particular day, I think you would be surprised at how much you depend on your body to produce enzymes to digest your meals and snacks.

Products of incompletely digested food molecules are absorbed into the blood through a process called the leaky gut syndrome. The immune system doesn't recognize these particulates, and treats them as the enemy, increasing the number of white blood cells. In order to digest the food, enzymes are then released from these cells, as well as from the lymphatic tissue and spleen, where they are stored. This is an abnormal function that the immune system shouldn't have to perform. If this condition becomes chronic, the body will create physical reactions, which are identified as food allergies. When the white blood cells are continually elevated due to a diet containing enzyme deficient foods, the immune system is weakened as the infection-fighting enzymes are now trying to digest food.

If you breathe environmental pollution, ingest toxins through the skin or eat cooked foods, enzymes are required to digest whatever is taken into the body. When inflammatory conditions show up, including food and environmental allergies, they may stem from enzyme deficiencies which began months before. Enzymes that are used up in the digestion of food cause the enzyme storage banks to become depleted. Viruses, bacteria and Candida yeast organisms can now have a field day because their exterminators are out feasting on food particles. Although the pancreas can produce digestive enzymes to digest the cooked food, it was not designed to work overtime, eventually losing the ability to make enzymes.

The size and weight of the pancreas will vary due to diet. The more this organ must work to compensate for enzyme deficient foods, the larger it gets. It must send messages to all parts of the body, looking for enzymes it can recycle. Changing the metabolic enzymes into digestive enzymes takes a lot of work for this organ. The enlargement may not harm the pancreas, but when it confiscates metabolic enzymes, it deprives the body by restricting the mechanics that every organ and cell needs to carry on its functions.

Raw foods provide their own enzymes, but in some instances they may not be released. Enzyme inhibitors are nature's way of protecting a plant. They keep enzymes inactive until such time as the seed, nut, grain or bean is ready for germination. This is why squirrels bury nuts. They instinctively know their nutrients are more bioavailable to the body when the enzymes are released, so they wait to eat them until just the right time. Beans, nuts and seeds are the types of raw foods that require enzyme supplementation, or you can wait until they begin sprouting to eat them.

An example of a popular food that contains enzymes inhibitors is the soybean. Many people who avoid meat and dairy want to assure themselves of adequate calcium and protein and therefore have switched to soy products. Although most recognize the nutritious advantage this bean gives you, raw soybeans do contain enzyme inhibitors which block the action of trypsin and other enzymes. These anti-nutrients are not completely deactivated during ordinary cooking, and those remaining may produce gastric distress, reduced protein digestion and chronic deficiencies in amino acid uptake. The protease inhibitors may have a beneficial side, as laboratory experiments have found they inhibit some types of cancer. In fermented soy (tempe, natto and miso) more of the enzyme inhibitors are deactivated and seem to pose no harm.

Trypsin inhibitors in the blood are growth depressants, not only affecting the hair, but also may restrict the normal development of children's bodies. This combination can lead to enlargement of the pancreas as the body tries to compensate by producing its own enzymes. A Fermented soy drink and fermented soy products have most of the enzyme inhibitors missing, because the bean has in effect begun to sprout. When soy products are cooked, a good many of the enzyme inhibitors may be killed, but the digestive enzymes die as well. Therefore if you decide to include cooked soy foods in your diet, take supplemental enzymes.

Soybeans are also high in phytates, an organic acid present in seed hulls, which blocks the intestinal tract uptake of essential minerals such as magnesium, calcium, iron and zinc. In persons with high iron, phytates will bind the iron in the intestines and may actually have the beneficial effect of inhibiting cancer. Non meat-eaters are more prone to deficiencies caused by phytates, because when soy products are consumed with meat, the mineral blocking effects of the phytates are reduced. Since soy is in so many food products, from baby formulas to additives (such as soy protein isolate and textured vegetable protein), you may want to do further research on both sides of the soy issue, before deciding on whether to ingest unfermented soy products.

Starch blockers, a recent diet fad, are actually enzyme inhibitors working on preventing starch from being assimilated. Although this may cause weight reduction, this process takes its toll on the pancreas, that must work overtime to provide enzymes to digest the starch. These blockers also cause a great quantity of enzymes to be excreted through the urine. The use of starch blockers can definitely shorten your lifetime through enzyme depletion. Food additives can also destroy enzymes, particularly catalase, found in almost all living cells of plants, animals and man. Catalase controls cell respiration, and sets up a barrier to virus infections, cancer and certain poisons.

Enzymes can't work alone, and most require the presence of vitamins and minerals known as co-enzymes, in order to do their work. For example, vitamins A, D, E, and K require fat for absorption and in order to be broken down, they need the enzyme, lipase. If this enzyme is missing, fat will not be digested and absorbed, and the vitamins will not be released. Water soluble vitamin B's and C, also help enzymes do their job. Vitamin C is necessary for the enzyme that helps make collagen, a major component of skin. Minerals and electrolytes are necessary because they are part of the enzyme structure. For instance, Zinc is part of more than two hundred enzymes and helps to metabolize food. It also is critical for the proper functioning of superoxide dismutase (S.O.D.), an enzyme that fights free radicals. So you see, that if enzymes are not present, the vitamins and minerals have no reason to be in the body.

Antioxidant enzymes are the first line of defense against free radical pathology. When the levels of free radicals are greater than the supply of antioxidant enzymes, the result is a free radical pathology (i.e., cancer, heart disease, etc.). Free radical damage to certain types of cells is irreversible. Heart muscle cells, nerve cells including brain cells, and certain sensor cells of the immune system cannot be replaced in the adult human. Damage to these cells must be prevented through use of S.O.D. along with Catalase, Glutathione Peroxidase and Methionine Reductase. These are enzymes that do not digest foods, but convert free radicals back into the original materials, oxygen and water. S.O.D. will not work without Catalase, and when combined, are effective free-radical converters that detoxify the body without the usual cleansing symptoms.

Glutathione Peroxidase consists of the amino acid glutathione and trace mineral selenium. It has been described as the best anti-aging agent naturally produced by the body. Free radical cross linking produces skin wrinkles. This enzyme is effective in approving skin appearance, shrinking moles, and making age spots disappear. It also helps chemically sensitive people control their allergies and build resistance to the effects of pollution. Methionine Reductase is an excellent enzyme to combat chemical poisoning from carbon monoxide, insecticides, air pollution, etc. It has detoxifying abilities of free radical toxins generated by mercury dental fillings.

Antioxidant enzymes work synergistically with other enzymes and co-factors. Isolated enzymes cannot duplicate this complex interaction. For this reason, the only way to insure that all antioxidant enzyme factors and co-factors are available for the body to use, is to provide the complete organic complex as it exists in living foods. Botanists have developed several unique strains of enzyme-rich supersprouts. They have demonstrated high levels of antioxidant enzymes, and have shown the remarkable ability to enhance the body's own production of antioxidant enzymes.

Enzymes can play a big role in anti-aging skin care. Trypsin, pancreatin and keratinase are used to break down and dissolve dead skin cells. Papain from young green papaya plants, has the ability to dissolve and digest old, debilitated or dead cells from the outer layer of the skin without harming the new cells. Green papaya enzymes assist the healing of uneven pigmentation, fine lines and brown spots by fighting free radical damage and boosting cell production. They are sometimes considered a natural alternative to Retin-A.

Research has turned up evidence that enzyme-replacement therapy can affect disease. The Bircher-Benner Sanitarium in

Switzerland noted great success with enzyme therapy for diabetes, ulcers, Graves disease asthma and arthritis. Impaired enzyme activity, especially lipase, may be the cause of certain cardiovascular diseases because lipase-stripped fats from cooking or processing, causes cholesterol deposits to form in the arteries. When lipase deficient fat meets hydrochloric acid in the human stomach, it is identified by the body in such a way that it is not digested. Thus, it may be improperly metabolized when it reaches the body tissue later.

Blood tests done in 1958 by L.O. Pilgeram of Stanford University demonstrated that there is a progressive decline in lipase in the blood of atherosclerosis patients with advancing middle and old age. Lipase, present in butter, unpasteurized milk, olives, flax seeds, poultry and animal fat is the enzyme found to be deficient in obese people. Indications show that when fats, whether animal or vegetable, are eaten along with their associated enzymes, no harmful effect on the arteries or heart results.

Arthritis has been called the 'cooked food' disease. After a study done in Manchester, England, scientists concluded that rheumatoid arthritis might be a deficiency disease arising from the inability of the body to deal adequately with protein digestion and metabolism. After 292 people were treated with enzymes, 264 showed improvement of various degrees. This type of success occurs over a long period of time and therefore is less attractive than pain killing drugs, but it also may solve the problem, permanently.

Enzymes are prescribed in medicine to digest blood clots and blocked vessels, clean up debris around infection, and are used for abscesses around catheters, valves and graphs. They are safe and effective for all people, including the elderly and babies. Researchers have found that enzymes can make leukemic cells return to normal cells and assist in the demise of cancer cells. Dr. Sherry Rogers saw a friend reduce a liver painfully swollen with cancer by using enzyme therapy. She discovered numerous reports of people who used enzymes to clear metastatic cancer after they were diagnosed as terminal. As in any therapy, massive doses of enzymes should be taken under advisement from a health practitioner.

Athletes are particularly susceptible to enzyme deficiency. The more they exercise, the more they eat and if they do not follow a raw food diet, they will use metabolic enzymes for digestion. This leaves fewer enzymes for organ and blood processes needed to insure the success of an athlete's performance.

Stress plays a big part in enzyme deficiency. Emotional problems, worry, fear, loneliness, even the stress of a physical problem, like getting dentures, can interfere with the secretion of digestive enzymes. This results in their decrease in tissue and fluids that can cause the skin to wrinkle and shrivel, hair to thin, muscles to sag, eyes to lose sparkle, and vitality to diminish. Stress and enzyme deficiency may be a contributing factor towards premature aging.

You can not get enough enzymes. There are no synthetic enzymes. Only living matter can product them and because plant enzymes work in a wider range of pH found in the digestive tract, they are better all around enzymes than animal-based types. Plant enzyme supplements help food to be assimilated in order to repair organs, glands, bones, muscles and nerves. Any excess is stored in the liver and the muscles. Like any addition to the body, tread lightly when first adding enzymes to your diet.

One of the jobs of enzymes is to act as house cleaners for the body. The addition of enzymes may cause an initial throwing off of toxins. This can result in intensification of symptoms, a "healing crisis." Some people get a skin rash as the toxins try to work their way out. As in any detoxification and rebuilding program, start out slowly and consult a health practitioner. Our advice is to consider taking enzymes every time you eat anything that is not raw. You will be surprised at how you can throw all of your antacids away. If you ever eat that big holiday dinner again and feel bloated and exhausted after the meal, you probably forgot to take your enzymes. Remember, you are not what you eat, but what you assimilate!

Recommended reading:
•*Enzyme Nutrition*, by Dr. Edward Howell
 Avery Publishing,

ESSENTIAL FATTY ACIDS

As we age, we want our quality of life to improve, or at least not deteriorate. Degenerative diseases that involve fat metabolism have been increasing throughout this century. In the early 1900's, people died of bacterial infections, poor surgical procedures, etc. In the near future it is expected that over half of American deaths will be caused by arterial, vascular and coronary heart disease. Fats have been implicated as one of the causes for this dilemma. The current craze is to eat fat-free. Low-fat diets may actually speed up the degenerative process because they are low in health-promoting essential fatty acids and contain high levels of damaging saturated and trans-fats.

Recent discoveries by Dr. Robert I-San Lin revealed that a prime suspect in the growth of cancer cells is a fat imbalance, not an overabundance of fats in general. Through experimentation he found that arachidonic acid, an essential fatty acid of the omega-6 variety, can actually promote cancer cell growth. Arachidonic acid is required for animals to grow. Normal cells divide and multiply up to a point at which stage they, in most cases, only replace those that have died. If this did not happen, our cells would engulf our bodies. When the omega-6 is not balanced by omega-3, these cells don't know when to stop. When those cells are cancerous, this becomes a dangerous condition.

Arachidonic acid only exists in animal bodies. When these animals eat feed containing large amounts of soybean and corn, their omega-6 production increases. People eating these animals may develop an essential fatty acid imbalance, unless they are also eating plants high in omega-3. During the last dozen years, garlic has been shown to modulate arachidonic acid metabolism, and it is suggested that it may modulate the cancer risk if essential fats are out of balance.

Fats come from animal and plant sources and usually take a solid form. Oils are produced mainly from plants and remain liquid. Fats and oils are both made of fatty acid molecules. Saturated fatty acid molecules are shaped like a straight line so they remain in a compact mass, staying hard at room temperature (butter). Monounsaturated fatty acids have a single "kink" in their molecular make up, which makes them more fluid (Olive and canola oils). These seem to play a beneficial role in the management of blood cholesterol, and therefore heart disease.

Polyunsaturated fatty acid molecules have two "kinks" that not only make them more fluid, but more likely to spoil easily (Safflower and corn oil). Super unsaturated fatty acids are molecules with three "kinks" and carry the most nutrients (black currant, flax, primrose oil). They also are most susceptible to spoilage and should be kept in a cool, dark place.

All of these fats are natural, but there's a fifth type of fat that's manufactured, and these are suspected to be the leading cause of health problems associated with fats. This process makes the fat more stable, and is popular with food manufacturers who do not have to refrigerate the oils. A chemical refining process is used to make this hydrogenated oil. Hydrogen is reacted with the liquid oil, using a catalyst such as nickel, zinc or copper. This substance becomes a smoky mass of grease, after which they de-gum the oils with phosphoric acid, which at the same time, removes several health promoting substances such as lecithin, chlorophyll and trace minerals. They are then bleached and re-colored to look like butter. This method converts healthy "cis-fatty acid" to a "trans-fatty acid."

The main sources of synthetic trans-fats are from margarine, shortening, deep fried foods cooked in partially hydrogenated high-heated oils, processed animal products and packaged foods containing hydrogenated oils (cookies, chips, bread, etc.). The head of Harvard School of Medicine, Dr. Walter Willet stated that the harmful effects of trans-fat laden margarine on the heart is connected to deaths from heart disease. Our bodies can handle an occasional ingestion of trans-fat foods, but over a lifetime, these unnatural substances accumulate and interfere with the normal biological chemistry of our bodies. They create corrupted organs and muscles, and cause cells to lose their DNA reproductive integrity, which promotes aging and degenerative disease.

Trans-fats can decrease testosterone production, promote pregnancy complications and contribute to low birth weight babies. They promote diabetes and cancer, alter the immune function and tax the liver's ability to process toxins. Researchers at the Harvard Medical School did a study of 85,000 female nurses over the course of eight years. They discovered that the women with the highest trans-fat intake had a 50% higher rate of heart attacks and coronary artery disease.

Trans-fats such as hydrogenated soybean and tropical palm kernel oil are solid at body temperature thereby remaining sticky and are likely to clog our arteries. They also interfere with prostaglandin production (hormone-like regulators in the blood) and kidney functions, as well as promote ulcers. Unnatural trans-fats disrupt the body's metabolism by changing the permeability of cells to let in viruses, toxins and parasites. This syndrome is called leaky gut. Cholesterol levels also reflect elevations in the bad LDL when trans-fats are consumed for as little as a three-week period. If this substance is eliminated from the diet, the cell's fluid membrane will be better able to transport and metabolize excess sugars, fats and toxins, and help to cleanse the body.

It is important to use oils in as natural a state as possible. This not only means refraining from using hydrogenated oil, but also choosing cold-extracted oils. Most mass market oils are refined, being obtained by chemical solvent extraction at a temperature of 500°F. These solvents may be carcinogenic and the high temperatures "kill" many of the nutrients. Expeller-pressed oils are produced through a chemical-free mechanical process which limits temperatures to 185°F. Cold pressed oils also use a mechanical process in which temperatures are restricted to 120° F., allowing more of the nutrients to remain intact. The higher the temperature used in the extraction process, the lower the nutrient quality of the oil. Refined olive oil loses over 100 volatile compounds that gives it a distinct taste. Oils should be labeled "cold pressed" or "virgin" for maximum quality. One of the best oils for health is virgin olive oil. It protects against heart disease and is implicated in cancer prevention. It also contributes to blood sugar control, essential for diabetics. Make sure olive oil is labeled "virgin" to be sure you are getting an unrefined nutritious product. ("Pure" labels are still a refined product.)

When we consume refined polyunsaturated oils on a regular basis, we can create an environment for cancer to develop. Immune system function is being suppressed by an imbalance in the ratio of omega-6 to omega-3 oils, thereby restricting the body's ability to fight disease. These essential fatty acids (EFAs) were discovered at the University of Minnesota by George and Mildred Burr in 1929. They cannot be made by the body, but must be taken in with food.

EFAs are the foremen in the body's workforce. They are required for the formation of prostaglandins which are hormone-like substances that tell cells when to divide or not to divide, when to take in nutrients, when to expel waste products, when to lay down bone or absorb bone, when to wake up or sleep, to feel pain, to form a clot, etc. Without prostaglandins, the body would be totally discombobulated. Without EFAs, prostaglandins would be on a permanent vacation. Essential fatty acid therapy should also include a broad spectrum of vitamins and minerals. The co-factors (see Appendix) of EFA metabolism are vitamins C, E, A, beta carotene, biotin, B3, B6 and the minerals Zinc and Magnesium.

Problems that can be associated with essential fatty acid deficiency are skin and airway membrane damage, suppression of the immune system, brittle nails, dry skin, hair loss, depression, ringing of the ears, cold intolerance, chronic pain, asthma, irritable bowel syndrome, heart disease, migraines and arthritis. If you experience any of these symptoms you may want to analyze your diet to see if you are lacking EFAs or are eating foods to create an EFA imbalance.

EFAs play a big part in maintaining the structure of the cells and of producing energy in the body. When they are not balanced, they compromise health. Omega-6 fatty acid (linoleic acid) is found in vegetable oils and bee pollen. In normal diets, it is consumed in great quantities and rarely a deficiency. Omega-3 (alpha-linolenic acid) is found in flax and fish oils predominantly, although trace amounts can be found in canola oil, soybean oil and walnut oil.

One of the best nutritional sources of omega-3 is flax. It can reverse the degenerative process. EFAs prevent heart disease by thinning the blood and removing cholesterol. They also normalize the immune system response by subtly affecting the production of prostaglandins and leukotrienes, two body chemicals made from fatty acids. One of the primary good side effects of taking flax is that it is an internal wrinkle cream. By providing moisture and necessary oils from the inside, the skin becomes softer and wrinkles seem to fill in and lessen.

Since we want to create a balance in essential fatty acids, adding flax to your diet is an easy fix. Flax can be purchased as oils, capsules, flaxmeal or you can grind your own flaxseed. Flax is a source of lignin, a plant compound that our body converts to lignan, anti-carcinogenic, antifungal. These are antiviral substances that we synthesize in our bowels when bacteria breaks down plant food in the digestive tract. All vegetables provide lignan precursors, but flax provides 800mg per gram as compared to only 8 mg per gram from other fiber sources. Flax fiber can protect against colon cancer and breast cancer by flushing excess estrogen and other carcinogens out of the body.

Gamma-linoleic acid (GLA) is identical to omega-3 fatty acids except for its bonding structure and therefore gives similar health benefits. GLA can be found in borage (24%), black currant (18%) and evening primrose oils (9%). If you eat saturated fats or refined vegetable oils, you may block the body's natural ability to create GLA from linoleic acids. Other GLA blockers are sugar, virus infections, dietary deficiencies and diabetes. Supplementation is absolutely necessary if you are not eating right, have liver problems, inflammatory disease or experience PMS.

Essential fatty acids should be an important part of your diet, especially if you exercise, as EFAs help the cells to recover from muscle use and overuse. They are needed by our glands to carry out the secretion of hormones and other regulating substances, and are essential to infant pre-natal and post-natal development. If you supplement your diet with omega-3 products, you will definitely see a change in the texture of your skin, and notice a reduction in the depth of lines in your face.

One very important reason for men to avoid trans-fats and balance EFAs is that baldness may be avoided. A report on the correlation between heart attacks and baldness, reveals that the gunk created by trans-fats adheres to both the arterial wall and hair follicles. This plaque builds up, smothering the hair and preventing it from getting oxygen. Thus hair actually stops growing because it is buried under layers of fatty goo. Once these layers are cleaned off and the trans-fats eliminated from the diet, dormant hair may actually emerge intact, or new growth will be regenerated. Predisposition to hair loss for "genetic" reasons may be diminished if men will avoid hats that make their head sweat, keep the scalp clean, and avoid trans-fat causing foods.

GREENS AND LIVE FOODS

Poisons in our environment known as free radicals damage the red blood cells, changing their shape from smoothly round to an irregular shape. This change of shape decreases the surface area that normally would rub against the capillary wall, causing the release of oxygen to the cells. This brings to mind the importance of antioxidants, which are substances that help to balance the body's love/hate affair with oxygen. Oxygen, though necessary for life, can also damage body tissue if present in areas that the body does not need it. Antioxidants prevent the oxidation of cells by excess oxygen. There are many antioxidants. The best ones are not only those that are absorbed into the blood, but those that are absorbed and utilized by each individual cell in the body. Many substances are absorbed into the blood and then excreted by the kidneys or the liver. Therefore they really have no action in the cells themselves. The more food-based these substances are, the more likely they will be used by the body.

Cereal grasses and green leafy vegetables. Since people are eating more and more cooked or processed meals, they are not getting the nutrients present in raw foods. Beneficial vitamins and minerals necessary for a youthful appearance and healthy body, are found in dark colored green vegetables. As we get older and nutritionally abuse our bodies, we are less resistant to degenerative disease. Part of staying young is to prevent the acceleration of this aspect of the aging process. Consuming raw greens or supplements will definitely keep time on your side.

Many years ago, Dr. G.H. Earp-Thomas, in his quest for duplicating an electrolyte formula, worked with wheat grasses. He discovered that the grasses contained a unique, electrical magnetic energy. The relatively high level of the electrical

61

energy force, transferred from the earth's magnetic field, is sent via these same live grasses. Walking on bare earth links us to this energy source. This aids immensely our body's magnetic, electrical "battery", so critically necessary for good health. Live plants transfer this energy from the earth; therefore, when you eat raw greens you receive the benefit of highly energized foods, necessary to keep you at your optimal best.

Green foods can also strengthen the immune system by providing the nutrients needed for the synthesis of the immune cells. Greens also contain an anti-peptic ulcer factor, protect our bodies from the effects of radiation, lower serum cholesterol, support healthy blood and circulation, as well as help maintain proper operation of the intestinal tract. They are nature's vitamin pill, providing C, A, iron, folic acid, protein, B12, K and calcium.

Dr. Benjamin Lau, M.D., Ph.D., from California's Loma Linda University Medical School found that barley grass, wheat grass and Chlorella are all potent stimulators of macrophages (cellular scavengers) which play a vital role in the immune system. When small quantities of these compounds are present, the macrophages produce powerful chemical substances that are known to kill bacteria, viruses and cancer cells. This may also be the reason that Japanese women, who include seaweed in their diet, have fewer incidents of breast cancer than their counterparts eating western-style meals.

Young barley leaves and wheat grass are good natural sources of chlorophyll, minerals (particularly high in calcium, magnesium and potassium), vitamins and enzymes needed for proper metabolism of our body cells. The Japanese claim that daily consumption of cereal grass juice helps reverse the aging process due to its high enzyme and anti-oxidant activity.

Harvesting cereal grasses at the right time is important, because they go through several stages as they grow. During each stage their chemical and nutritional profiles vary widely. In the early stages, they store large amounts of chlorophyll, vitamins and proteins. If cut or eaten at this stage, they will grow again. During the next stage (jointing) the grass begins to form a stem which is the peak of a cereal plant's vegetative development. After the jointing stage, the stem forms branches and continues to grow, increasing cellulose levels while decreasing chlorophyll, protein and vitamins. Once this stage is reached the plant should not be harvested until it produces seed because it will not regenerate itself. It is optimal to harvest cereal grass during the first stage, to reap maximum nutritional benefits from the growing cycle. Dried barley grass juice harvested at the proper time, can have five times the iron in spinach, seven times the vitamin C in oranges and an abundance of bioflavonoids that can slow down cellular oxidation (aging). When selecting supplements, question suppliers to determine if the harvesting criteria have been met.

Consuming greens can help add healthy years to your life, and increase your resistance to disease. A report in the American Journal of Clinical Nutrition (41:32-36), indicates that elderly people are the least likely group to die from cancer, if their diet contains an abundance of green and yellow vegetables. Cereal grasses contain strong anti-cancer agents such as the anti-oxidant vitamins E and A, Zinc, and the trace mineral selenium. Anti-tumor effects in animals have also been demonstrated by an intake of Chlorella, Kelp, and chlorophyll.

Studies show that several green vegetables provide anti-mutagenic protection from a number of cancer-causing chemicals. This activity is found to be proportional to the concentration of chlorophyll in the vegetables (darker green is better). Chlorophyll has been called concentrated sun power. It is the outcome of photosynthesis and in wheat grass juice, accounts for 70% of the solid content. Chlorophyll is to the plant as blood is to the animals. Long known only as a disinfectant, chlorophyll is a natural blood builder, and also heals wounds by stimulating repair of damaged tissues and inhibiting growth of bacteria. It is effective in speeding the healing of peptic ulcers, diseases of the colon, and treating pancreatitis and kidney stones.

Chlorophyll has been known to cure acute infections of the respiratory tract, and controls halitosis and oral diseases. This antioxidant has even been shown to nullify the effects of a variety of environmental and food substances (such as cigarette smoke, diesel fumes, coal dust, and fried beef), which are known to cause mutation. It can actually be more effective than vitamin A, C or E antioxidants. Chlorophyll therapy provides an excellent alternative to drug therapy, because repeated tests have shown it produces virtually no toxic side effects.

One major advantage that chlorophyll provides to the body is its ability to help alkalize the pH in the blood. When pH is too acid, free radicals reign, anti-oxidants are immobilized and therefore cannot do their job of attacking invaders. The body tends to buffer this acidity with sodium, causing stomach upset, and also calls upon its next buffer, calcium, which is drawn from the bones and placed into the blood. Calcium lodges in the bloodstream and sets the stage for arthritis. Therefore, it is absolutely necessary to add chlorophyll foods to your diet to help balance the pH.

When adding greens to your diet, you may consider cereal grasses and seaweed along with organic dark leafy vegetables. Pesticides are not beneficial to health, therefore whenever possible, insist on organic food and/or supplements. Dehydrated cereal grasses such as wheatgrass and barley grass contain highly concentrated amounts of necessary nutrients, and may be the answer to high-paced lifestyles, where more concentrated stores of energy are required.

Vegetables for protein. A fact little understood by meat and dairy consumers is that vegetarianism does not necessarily lead to protein deficiency. A grain and vegetable-centered diet, including wheat or barley grass, may actually result in a higher intake of protein than a meat based diet. Dehydrated cereal grasses contain 25% protein, whereas milk (3%), eggs (12%) and steak (16%) are all lower! Even bee pollen contains five to seven times more protein than beef, eggs, and cheese of equal weight. Adequate protein is necessary for the formation of essential compounds including antibodies, hormones, neurotransmitters and enzymes, and for the growth of all tissues and replacement of damaged tissues. It also is an important source of food energy and helps maintain the electrolyte/water balance and the body's pH.

Vegetable proteins have been considered incomplete (not containing *all* 20 amino acids) and therefore cannot be optimally used by the body like animal food proteins. Cereal grass is different, according to Pines, manufacturers of wheat and barley grass supplements, claiming they contain all the essential amino acids in amounts that make its protein usable in the body. From a protein standpoint, cereal grass must be an important part of all non-animal based diets

Chlorella and sea vegetables. In addition to cereal grasses and dark greens, sea vegetables, algae and Chlorella play an important role in micronutrient assimilation. Years of intense farming methods have leached adequate levels of micronutrients (trace elements essential for normal growth and development) from our soils, leaving the foods grown on those soils, deficient. When micronutrients are added back into a diet, people often find that in addition to having more energy overall, immunity is boosted. This results in an increased ability to cope with stress and to ward off infection. In addition, chronic allergies and asthma may disappear, seemingly overnight. An additional benefit to the increase of micronutrients is that the skin becomes clear and bright, hair becomes thicker and shinier, and fingernails grow longer and stronger. Micronutrient consumption has also been linked to decreases in some of the symptoms of PMS, and cystic breast disease.

Besides improving the condition of already existing hair, micronutrient supplementation has also been responsible for hair re-growth and restoring pigmentation to gray hair. A documented case history describes a young girl in Connecticut who suffered from alopecia (baldness). A noted children's hospital prescribed different shampoos and when they had no effect, the doctors said her condition was stress related and gave up on her. A hairdresser suggested she add SOURCE micronutrients to her diet, and within four months hair started growing back on her head. In a test case, a horse was give micronutrients for warts and a poor hoof condition. What they didn't expect was for his gray hair to turn color again as a result of the treatment. This gives a clue to the fact that some cases of gray hair may be attributed to lack of essential nutrients in our diets.

Sea vegetables have received a reprieve from man's destruction (so far). They are abundant in minerals, for example, Kelp which is high calcium, iodine, potassium, and magnesium. It is also a good source of Vitamin C. Kelp sparks vital enzyme reactions, and increases thyroid metabolism so it may be effective in weight control. Kelp has been used in folk medicine to treat respiratory, gastrointestinal and genitourinary problems and has been shown to lower blood pressure and cholesterol. In animal tests, Dr. Jane Teas found that feeding rats with kelp significantly delayed and reduced the development of breast cancer induced by chemical carcinogens. It is speculated that kelp contains compounds which may counteract carcinogens or cancer-producing substances, and it may do so by modulating the immune system.

Chlorella is a single cell, globular green, water borne algae, that is the largest selling health food supplement in Japan. It is rich in chlorophyll, minerals, vitamins A, B3, B2, B6, pantotheic acid, folic acid, choline, biotin, lypoic acid, nucleic acid and other substances that provide various biological effects. It is high in protein (see chart), has 800 times as much vitamin C as milk, and is reported to have the ability to stimulate the immune system. It isn't the amount of protein in Chlorella that makes a difference in our health, but the kind of protein it is. Chlorella supplies all the essential amino acids in good balance, and is thus an excellent whole food in itself.

Dr. Bernard Jensen in *Chlorella, Gem of the Orient*, states that "Dr. Benjamin Frank, author of *The No-Aging Diet*, suggests that human RNA/DNA production slows down as people age, resulting in lower levels of vitality and increased vulnerability to various diseases. When we eat foods rich in DNA and RNA it protects our own cellular nucleic acids, allowing the cell wall to function efficiently. As a result, the cell remains clean and well-nourished." Dr. Michinori Kimura found that Chlorella consists of ten percent RNA, and three percent DNA, which would make it the most concentrated source of nucleic acids in the world, being seventeen times more concentrated than sardines, the next best source.

Protein comparison per 100 grams	
CHLORELLA	67
BEEF	24-27
FISH	18-29
CHICKEN	24
WHEAT	13
EGGS	13
RICE	3
POTATOES	3

The Chlorella is a 2½ billion year-old single-cell algae that doesn't die, but instead reproduces itself into four new Chlorella cells. If we could teach the cells in our bodies to multiply rather than age and die, we could definitely prolong life. Chlorella Growth Factor (CGF) promotes this cell multiplication and prevents disease by repairing and renewing organs, glands and tissues in the body. Experiments have shown that CGF promotes faster-than-normal growth without any adverse side effects.

Chlorella cells are very tiny organisms, grown in special culture pools and should not be confused with spirulina which is a multi-cell plant with larger cells that are harvested from lakes and ponds. Chlorella has been an effective treatment for gastric and duodenal ulcers, lowering cholesterol and blood pressure, fighting cancer, warding off cold germs, aiding in intestinal peristalsis, and has been used in treatment of incurable wounds. It combats the effects of aging, strengthens the immune responses and promotes growth in young children and animals.

A thirty-eight year old man who was suffering from high blood pressure and impotence, among a lot of other health problems, was told by his doctor to increase his intake of greens. For this patient who disliked vegetables, the doctor recommended Kyo-Green®, a powder containing Chlorella, Laminaria (kelp), young barley leaves and wheat grass (a high source of chlorophyll). Within one week the man's blood pressure had returned to normal. Within two weeks, his stamina and his sexual potency returned, and many other symptoms which he had considered just a part of life, disappeared. The power of greens and seaweed can definitely make a difference.

Another potent green food is Hawaiian Spirulina, considered one of the premium green superfoods. It provides exceptionally concentrated nutrition in a whole food form our bodies can very easily digest and absorb. This concentrated whole food source of phyto-nutrients can supply the body with a rich mixture of carotenoids, chlorophyll, enzymes, complete vegetarian protein, B- vitamins and a newly discovered anti-viral compound called calcium spirulan.

Blue green algae, one of 50,000 species of algae, seaweed and plankton, is also a nutrient-dense food and only a small amount is necessary to supply the body with a little of almost every nutrient that it needs. It provides biologically active vitamins, minerals, trace elements, amino acids, simple carbohydrates, enzymes, fatty acids, carotenoids, and chlorophyll. Its protein content is of a type called glycoproteins, which is more easily broken down and assimilated by the body than lipoproteins found in vegetables and meat.

Algae and sea vegetables are used for healing purposes throughout the world, and should be part of everyone's diet. All green vegetables and cereal grasses should be consumed raw to maximize bioavailablity of the nutrients. If you prefer to cook your greens, make sure you take your plant enzyme supplement.

Micronutrients from the sun. Two thousand years before written history began, a civilization known as the Sumerians learned how to harness the power of the sun. With this knowledge they transformed a land of dust and mud into a great civilization whose honored and ancient knowledge became the foundation for the great cultures of Egypt, Greece, Rome and the western world. Their technology acknowledged that plants are a superior source of antioxidants, and considered by some as the ultimate solar battery. They knew that complex chemical reactions convert fuel sources from the sun to the primary energy compound, for use in our muscle cells. This compound is known today as adenosine triphosphate (ATP). Harvested plants provide our cells with energized food so they can make this ATP, which is the only compound known to provide life force to all living things. The result is that our cells are nourished and now have the ability to slow the aging process, as well as increase genetic efficiency.

New technology has found a way to provide the proteins and nucleotides direct from the plants to the cells without a conversion process. Rather than providing cells with glucose so they can make ATP, we are providing them with the ATP directly. This process allows a free flow of life energy, which is called

"Superlattice". This pattern is known to be the same pattern of order in our mitochondria, the energy factory in our cells. This new system of Bio-Physics is creating a basis for a higher order of life. Visualize that the DNA is like a flashlight with the proteins functioning as the battery and the genes functioning as the bulb. If the battery (proteins) run down, the bulb (genes) will go out or turn off. Conversely, if you recharge the proteins (the battery) the genes (the bulb) will come back on and function again. The more you charge the protein, the better and more normally functional the genes will become. This new process becomes the facilitator to recharge our cellular structure.

The proteins, when charged, reject free radicals. This results in less damage to the internal organs, a reduction or elimination of genetic disease, and prevents cells from dying (anti-aging). This can be accomplished by transforming concentrated organic fruit juices, honey and teas through a solar distillation process to change the sun's power into chemical energy that can be used by the body. This is 24th century nuclear cellular technology available now, that the Sumarians depicted in their ancient picture writings. It is truly medicine of the past that can turn back the clock for our future generations.

Recommended Reading:
•*Chlorella, Jewel of the Far East*, By Bernard Jensen, Ph.D.
•*Wheatgrass, Nature's Finest Medicine*, Steve Meyerowitz
 Sprout House Publishing, 1998

NATURAL TREATMENTS.

Aloe. Aloe vera is a wonderful plant that you can grow in your home. Widely known for its topical use for specific skin conditions such as burns, insect bites, acne, cuts and eczema, aloe also can be beneficial if taken internally. Aloe supplements, including aloe drinks, activate the immune cells, and in particular, activate the scavenging macrophages and neutrophils which carry out the clean-up operations to rid our body of toxic waste. Aloe activates the healthy cells into a growth and replication phase, accompanied by much protein synthesis and the general build-up of tissue constituents. These 'activated' cells can now increase the detoxification process, and facilitate support of the immune system. Ridding our body of excess debris is extremely important if we are to stay young.

Almonds. Almonds contain the right kind of fats, monounsaturated and some polyunsaturated fats, which help lower the bad cholesterol (LDL) while not interfering with the HDL (good cholesterol). They also don't contribute to weight gain. Almonds are loaded with protein, fiber, calcium, magnesium, potassium, vitamin E and other antioxidants and phytochemicals. In a study of 45 men and women with high cholesterol, those on an almond based diet for four weeks showed greater decreases in total cholesterol and LDL levels, compared with those on an olive oil based diet, as reported in the Journal of American College of Nutrition 17:285-90, 1998.

One ounce of almonds contains 35% of the daily value of vitamin E that is thought to protect the body's cells from damaging free radicals. Two phytochemicals, quercetin and kaempferol, have been shown to inhibit the growth of lung, prostate and breast tumors in laboratory studies. Almond milk and almond butter are available if you don't like eating nuts. If

71

you find nuts create gas in your stomach, try taking digestive enzymes when you eat them.

Help from our friends, the bees. Bees have been helping people for centuries. They collect pollen from flowers and deposit it in the honeycomb cell where it is concentrated, becoming a high source of nutrients. RNA and DNA are found in abundant quantities in bee pollen as well as rutin, which strengthens capillaries. It has been suggested that it can control the runaway growth of cancer cells, reduce alcohol craving, increase IQ and the powers of concentration. High in lecithin, bee pollen also contributes to the increase in brain function. Taken before and during allergy season, it has been effective in preventing the onset of symptoms. When purchasing bee pollen products, research their drying process. Heating or microwaving, a popular method, kills beneficial organisms, therefore natural drying and/or freezing is best.

Another bee 'product' is royal jelly. This is the white, milky substance produced in the glands of worker honeybees to feed the queen and help her grow 40-60% larger than the other bees. Royal jelly contains all of the B-complex vitamins, A,C,D, and E, minerals, enzymes, hormones, eighteen amino acids as well as antibacterial and antibiotic components. It is known to aid asthma, liver disease, pancreatitis, insomnia, stomach ulcers, kidney disease, bone fractures and skin disorders. It aids the immune system and produces an age-retarding, longevity-enhancing effect.

Propolis is the bees' natural defense against bacteria, fungi and viruses. It can act against viruses where current antibiotics are ineffective, by preventing them from reproducing. Since natural antibiotics from flavonoids, such as propolis, possess a cellular structure similar to the human body, they may be much more effective than existing antibiotics such as penicillin and streptomycin. Propolis also is an antioxidant free-radical scavenger and can stimulate the body's own immune system to resist disease. According to John Diamon, M.D., president of the International Academy of Preventive Medicine, propolis may be the most strengthening to the thymus, of all the natural supplements he tested. It can be used topically for healing wounds and infections, treating ulcers, controlling cancer and for sore throats, coughs, colds, sinusitis and tonsillitis.

Of course, for healing bee products we can't forget to mention honey. If it is unprocessed and made in an organic environment, it can be used topically as a dressing agent in surgical infections, burns and wound infections, and is an old folk remedy for stomach upset, sore throats and as a more healthful sugar substitute

Bioflavonoids. Referred to by some as vitamin P, bioflavonoids are the largest group of antioxidants that fight the free radicals in our system. These free radicals can cause cellular damage that has been shown to be a contributing factor in a myriad of diseases. Bioflavnoids can help the body protect itself against these free radicals. They also help alleviate the symptoms of asthma, assist in preventing build up of arterial plaque and lowering cholesterol, enhance capillary and vein strength to reduce male sexual dysfunction, protect connective tissue, and reduce bruising.

Essential oils. Essential oils have been used since the beginning of recorded history. They were the origins of medicine as liquid antiseptics, and the origins of perfume, due to their concentrated pure powerful aromas. The rejuvenating properties of essential oils for cell tissue and for mental-emotional health has been well known from the Egyptians to current holistic health practitioners. When using essential oils, care should be given to choose pure, unadulterated high-grade products to gain the maximum benefit of its cell-rejuvenation abilities. They should be mixed with a high-grade base oil such as organic golden jojoba, before applying on the skin.

Aromatherapy is the therapeutic use of essential oils. Frankincense, Sandalwood, Geranium and rose are excellent for rejuvenation facial gels and body massage blends. Hippocratic prescription for health was to take a scented bath or aromatic massage each day. Today we can accomplish this through using straight essential oils for inhalation, or by blending with a base oil for use in a bath or as a massage oil. As with most external therapies, essential oils should not be taken internally nor used on the skin without first diluting.

Growth Hormone. According to Dr. H.A. Davis, author of *Feeling Younger with Homeopathic HGH*, "when our long bone growth is completed between ages 20 and 25, the brain's pituitary and immune system lose their motivation. Instead of going to a balanced level, Human Growth Hormone (HGH) begins to decrease steadily, and signs of aging appear. These can include wrinkles, thinning hair, diminishing eyesight, failing sexual performance, cholesterol imbalance, poor memory, gray hair, sleep difficulties, emotional instability and lack of muscle tone."

Studies show that growth hormone continues to decline as we age. One of the theories for this is that the internal organs develop scar tissue from a lack of nutrients, diseases, nitrites, smoking, excessive alcohol intake, surgery, cholesterol, etc. Scar tissue formed in the liver and pituitary (the main source of growth hormone), will impede the production of growth hormone.

For years, HGH supplementation has been available through expensive injections, and more recently through effective supplements of "secretagogues" that "wake up" the endocrine glands. Medical studies show growth hormone supplementation works better when taken at frequent intervals and in smaller amounts. Homeopathic forms of growth hormone ingestion follow this parameter. Not only are they effective, but they are economical, and don't come with a list of side effects. Homeopathic forms of growth hormone also are thought to penetrate scar tissue better that other forms, and therefore become more effective at improving the production of growth hormone in the glands.

While most physicians today are familiar with recognizing and treating hormone deficiencies, there is generally a disregard for the complex interaction that all hormones have with one another. Insulin is a hormone that greatly affects the secretion and response to estrogen, growth hormone, progesterone, melatonin and testosterone. The aging process results in a declining ability to manage insulin and other hormones. If insulin is not regulated, much higher doses of estrogen must be used to attain the desired response. The methods by which human growth hormone (HGH) interacts, include insulin regulation and control of blood glucose, which are both essential to growth hormone release. Excess insulin and blood sugar inhibit the ability of hormones like estrogen and testosterone to get into the cell and perform their function. The response to the sex hormones is enhanced with growth hormone therapy.

The benefits of growth hormone supplementation can be one or any of the following: improved stamina, sounder sleep, increase in energy, improved muscle tone, stronger nail growth, better digestion, weight loss, enhanced sexual function, increase in strength, improved mental processes, hair growth, less pain, reduction of wrinkles, diminished cellulite, eyesight improvements, emotional stability. These are reasons enough to try supplemental growth hormone.

Many new diet and growth hormone enhancing products contain L-Arginine as an ingredient. A word of caution: any person suffering from any form of the herpes virus, including chronic cold sores or shingles, should use caution when considering these products as L-Arginine has been clinically shown to stimulate the growth of the Herpes Virus.

Homeopathic. Homeopathic remedies treat illness by stimulation of the body's own healing response. They are prepared from natural substances: plant, mineral and animal. Homeopathic treatment operates under the premise that the same natural substances that cause a set of symptoms when given to a healthy individual in large quantities, can also stimulate a sick individual to get better if given in tiny amounts.

Every disease which afflicts the human race indicates a lack of some inorganic constituent of the body. Biochemical supplements given in small quantities help to restore that which is missing. Flower remedies tend to work on the emotional level, from which many of our ailments originate. Since illness can be influenced positively or negatively by a person's mental state, flower remedies may head sickness off at the pass. There are numerous books that describe these alternative methods in detail, so we won't re-invent the wheel, but we have listed various homeopathic remedies later in this book under the heading for specific illnesses.

Lecithin. If lecithin were a drug instead of a natural food, our doctor would probably be prescribing it as beneficial to the brain, nervous system, cardiovascular system, liver and other vital parts of the body. Lecithin is a phospholipid, a fat-like substance that is produced in the liver, and is also present in some foods such as egg yolks, fish, wheat germ, nutritional yeast and soy. The most widely known use of lecithin is in decreasing harmful cholesterol levels by preventing it from depositing on arterial linings.

Lecithin also is known to help in the recovery of memory loss and improving brain activity. According to studies at the Massachusetts Institute of Technology (MIT), lecithin improved memory not only in the aged, but in people in their thirties as well. In 1975 scientists at MIT discovered that lecithin choline has a prompt effect on the brain's ability to make an important chemical (acetylcholine) for nerve signal transmission. This is taken up by the brain directly (crossing the blood brain barrier), causing an immediate effect on brain chemicals. Scientific studies indicate that we can repress those age-related brain changes by long-term use of lecithin supplements.

Phytochemicals.   Foods contain hundreds of naturally occurring compounds, called phyto-chemicals. Although they have no nutritional value, these organic chemical substances are found naturally in plants. Garlic is one of these and we have explained its benefits elsewhere in this book. Its primary attribute is that it has the ability to defend cells from free-radical damage, and protect the nervous system and the heart by lowering blood cholesterol and blood triglycerides. Iycopene is a phytochemical that causes tomatoes to appear red in color. This also is a high antioxidant, especially when the fruit is heated. Iycopene is also found in watermelon, pink grapefruit, shellfish (crab and lobster) and guava.

Citrus fruits also contain high amounts of phyto-chemicals. They contain the anti-cancer properties of terpenes, limonins and flavonoids. Tea is another extremely good source of phytochemicals coming in the form of catechin and flavonols. They help reduce the conditions that cause heart disease, some types of cancers and strokes. Other natural occurring substances are plant sterols. These have the ability to lower cholesterol, although levels are normally too small from normal dietary consumption. They are found in vegetable oils, wheat, corn and rye. Progress is under way to manufacture a fat-soluble derivative of plant sterol as a food additive, to give higher concentrations that can be beneficial in affecting cholesterol levels.

Shark liver oil. This is an old Norwegian folk remedy used traditionally by fishermen for healing wounds and irritations of the respiratory tract and alimentary canal. It contains alkylglycerols (AKG), squalamine and squalene. AKG's are a group of fats know to bolster the immune system, enhance response to colds and allergies, accelerate wound healing and suppress tumor growth. Shark liver oil is a medicinal supplement and should be used after consultation with a health practitioner.

Tachyon. The disorganization of the subtle organizing energy fields (SOEFs) is called positive entropy or aging. The increased organizing of the SOEFs is called negative entropy or youthing. When the SOEFs are energized, improvement of cell function, youthing and improved health occurs. When SOEFs are depleted of energy, we get an increase in the aging process. Nutrients are defined as that which energizes the SOEFs: sunlight, oxygen, live organic foods and tachyon energy.

Tachyon is a theoretical subatomic particle that moves faster than the speed of light with real energy, but no mass. It is known as the life force energy. When it is blocked, our electrical system can short circuit and prevent healing. By using SOEFs including Tachyonized products, we can clear such blocks. Using a darkfield microscope to perform a live blood analysis, confirmation can be determined as to the benefit of these SOEFs, including tachyons, on live blood characteristics and activity. For the first time in history, we have scientific methods of restructuring certain materials at the sub-molecular level that then become antennae to attract and focus usable biological energy, i.e., Tachyon energy.

Recommended reading:
•*Feeling Younger with Homeopathic HGH,* Dr. H.A. Davis,
 Safe Goods Publishing
•*Growth Hormone, The Methuselah Factor,* Dr. L.E. Dorman,   James Jamieson, Valerie Marriott
 Safe Goods Publishing

PLANTS ASSURE LONGEVITY

Since the days of the Old Testament, humans have been tapping the enormous healing power of plants. Multi-billion dollar drug companies have not ignored the importance of herbs, with one-third of all prescription drugs sold in the United States being herbal extracts. Vincristine, a potent anti-cancer drug for childhood leukemia is made from the periwinkle plant and Digitalis, a common heart medicine is made from the foxglove plant. Folk remedies have included penicillin from moldy bread, aspirin naturally occurring in white willow and even quinine used for malaria, found in the Cinchona bark of the rain forests.

For thousands of years, the leaves of the ginkgo tree have been recognized for their benefits as a geriatric remedy. The most interesting and important relate to vascular disease, brain function, impotency, asthma and inflammation. By improving circulation, Ginkgo is a powerful treatment for restoring and boosting memory. A recent study published in a major scientific journal shows that an extract of this ancient botanical, success-fully restored erections to impotent men. In Sweden, blueberry extract and its drug name Pecarin, is used in the treatment of di-arrhea. Cranberries have long been known to alleviate urinary tract infections. Unfortunately, these and many other natural remedies cannot be patented, restricting their monetary viability for medical usage.

Herbs are concentrated foods, whole essences, with the ability to address both the symptoms and causes of a problem. They are foundational nutrients, working through the glands, to nourish the body's deepest basic elements. Balance is the key to using herbal nutrients for healing, with each person reacting differently. Herbs work better in combination than they do alone, and results from herbs may not be immediate. A rule of thumb states that you need one month of healing for every year of the illness. People wishing to find alternatives to drugs have investigated herbs, foods, as well as homeopathic, biochemical and flower remedies.

Chinese herbs have been used in healing for over 4,000 years. Balancing body, mind and spirit is the core of Traditional Chinese Medicine which combines the healing power of plants with the energy they release for specific conditions (similar to homeopathics). There are many herbal treatments for specific illness, as indicated later in this book. In this chapter, we will list our special choices and those we consider highly effective.

Garlic. They say you can tell an Italian by the garlic on his/her breath, but you can bet they are a lot healthier because of it. For over 5,000 years, garlic has been used in health care, mostly in the pure or raw bulb state. As far back as 1500 B.C., the Egyptians used garlic as an effective remedy for many ailments, including heart problems and tumors. It has long been considered a heart remedy in Ayurvedic medicine. Garlic has been purported to have healing power in the treatment of hypertension, arthritis, heavy metal poisoning, constipation and athlete's foot.

In the last 20 years, over 1800 scientific papers have been published on various aspects of garlic research. This magnificent food has the ability to decrease the levels of "bad" cholesterol, while raising the levels of "good" cholesterol. The Danish and Russians have used garlic for centuries, for coughs and colds. Grandmothers have been telling us to gargle with garlic to relieve a sore throat, or to apply garlic juice to ward off wound infections. Garlic is a natural antibiotic.

A study by the People's Republic of China reported residents of Cangshan County had a lower death rate due to stomach cancer than those living in the county of Qixia. They discovered that the Cangshan County residents regularly ate 20 grams of garlic per day, whereas the Qixia residents ate very little. (The reasoning behind the success of garlic in cancer prevention was attributed to the levels of nitrites in the gastric juices of the residents. Nitrites are the precursors of carcinogens. The Cangshan residents who ate garlic had lower levels of nitrites thereby inhibiting the growth of cancer.) Dr. Jinzhou Liu, a Chinese biochemist from Penn State University, proved that Kyolic® Aged Garlic Extract™ was more effective than Vitamin C in preventing nitrosamines from forming in laboratory experiments. Nitrosamines are one of the world's most potent known carcinogens.

Garlic has been thought of as a miracle cure. It is effective against forms of Staph, Strep, Bacillus and Salmonella and scores of other infectious agents. It is antibacterial, antifungal, antiviral and antiparasitic. Dr. Albert Schweitzer had success using it to treat typhus, cholera and typhoid. In China, eleven patients who had crypto-coccal meningitis were given Garlic extract orally and by injection. All eleven people recovered from this normally fatal disease.

In one study, ten AIDS patients were given Kyolic® liquid garlic extract for ten weeks while their normal natural killer cells and the helper/suppressor ratios in their immune systems were monitored. These readings were abnormal at the beginning of treatment, but by the end of the time period, six of seven patients had normal killer cell activity and four of seven patients had an improved killer/suppressor ratio. They also had a reduction in AIDS related symptoms including diarrhea, candidiasis, and genital herpes. This study was presented at the Fifth International Conference on AIDS in Montreal, Quebec, Canada in 1989,

In a 1973 experiment, nine people under the direction of pathologist Dr. Tariq Abdullah, tested the effect of garlic on natural killer cells against tumor cells. Three groups of volunteers were instructed to either avoid garlic, or take large doses of raw garlic or aged garlic extract. At the end of three weeks, blood samples were taken to determine how active each volunteer's natural killer cells were. The group taking raw garlic found their cells killed 139 percent more tumor cells than the group taking no garlic. The aged garlic extract group killed 159 percent more tumor cells than those of the control group.

Inasmuch as melanoma of the skin is so widespread throughout the United States, researchers at UCLA began using Aged Garlic Extract™ to treat this disease, finding that it suppresses the growth of cancer cells. Dr. Hoon says aged garlic extract may be the perfect modality for the prevention of melanoma. Troubled by the rapid rise in the number of new bladder cancer cases each year (more than 50,000), West Virginia researchers led by Dr. Donald Lamm found that Aged Garlic Extract™ reduced the tumor growth and according to Dr. Lamm, suggested that it will prove to be an extremely effective form of immunotherapy.

By now, you should be convinced that garlic is basic to good health and longevity. It can protect against pollution, radiation and even stress, kill many forms of harmful microbes and strengthen a person's immunity. Garlic may also have great potential for retarding aging, since it inhibits peroxidation, a natural process that is believed to be part of the cause of aging. The membranes of our cells in our bodies must be soft and flexible to keep us in optimum health. Peroxidation causes these cells to be stiff and inflexible and can lead to blood vessel damage and inhibition of food nutrients, all qualities that lead to premature aging and disease. The unique process involved in the aging of garlic inhibits this peroxidation process.

Garlic contains numerous minerals and vitamins, including A, B1 and C, calcium, magnesium, iron, copper, zinc, selenium, potassium chloride, germanium (enhances the immune system), sulfur compounds and various amino acids. Garlic increases the body's ability to assimilate thiamine by enhancing its absorption. Thiamine is a key part of the enzyme which acts beneficially on liver cells. Garlic is also effective in the treatment of lead, mercury, cadmium and arsenic poisoning, as its sulfur compounds bind these heavy metals facilitating excretion from the body. The major heavy metals, such as cadmium, lead and mercury, weakens our resistance to cancer, destroy morale and tax the immune system, leading to other diseases. Aged Garlic Extract™ has shown to increase the glutathione in the liver, thus helping the body to rid itself of pesticides, chemicals and toxins. Garlic is not just for people approaching mid-life who want to avoid illness; it is beneficial for everyone. Even if you don't like the taste of garlic, supplements can do the job equally as well, or even better.

<u>Allicin and media hype.</u> Although garlic has many beneficial properties, this wonderful herb is sometimes rejected because of its socially-scorned odor. "Allicin, the odoriferous chemical formed when a garlic clove is cut or bruised is not important at all," says Dr. Herbert Peirson, a consultant formerly with the U.S. National Cancer Institute. "Allicin is highly unstable and degrades instantly in processing, when exposed to heat, oxygen, light, proteins or changes in acidity," he explains. "It is not crucial to any of garlic's biological activities, which is good, because allicin is also toxic and can kill cells."

For years it was assumed that allicin was the effective component in garlic. Thanks to modern technology, we now know that this is not the case. The latest study by the Nobel Prize Chemistry Department of the University of California at Irvine, tested garlic products claiming to contain allicin. In October 1995 they proved conclusively that these claims are false. In 1990, Dr. Osamu Imada, speaking at the First World Congress on Garlic, indicated that allicin is one of the major harmful compounds in raw garlic and when garlic is aged, its toxicity is greatly reduced.

Research is discovering that aged garlic extract is very therapeutic, due to the fact that aging renders the garlic odorless and less irritating to the stomach. Aged garlic extract is standardized with S-allyl cysteine (SAC), a water-soluble sulfur-containing amino acid. The benefits of SAC have shown that it lowers serum cholesterol and triglycerides. Rather than degrading cholesterol, aged garlic extract appears to interfere with its synthesis better than other forms of garlic supplements. The aging of garlic enhances the activity of detoxifying anti-oxidant enzymes in our cells (S.O.D., Catalase, Glutathione), which triggers the immune system to ward off free radicals. Unless the cells in our body do the killing, we can never recover from the onslaught of diseases.

Studies have indicated that aged garlic extract helps combat infectious disease by strengthening the immune system. Research has determined that garlic actually attracts immune cells to the tissue. Aged garlic extract has been seen to inhibit Candida albicans growth, actually hastening the removal of these cells from the blood circulation. In one study, Aged Garlic Extract™ was even found to enhance the effectiveness of an influenza vaccine, and when used alone was found to be as effective as the vaccine.

Rhodiola Rosea. This herb is known as golden root and arctic root. Found naturally in the northern regions of Siberia and other arctic locations, Rhodiola Rosea detoxifies the liver, allowing the body to experience a more thorough cleansing. It also burns fats during periods of heavy exercise, instead of burning the body's principle energy carrying compound, adenosine triphosphate (ATP). This provides more rapid recovery from athletic endeavors, and also helps in weight reduction without depleting energy levels, a normal side-effect of weight loss programs. Rhodiola Rosea has adaptogenic properties, which is a natural plant substance that increases the body's resistance to disease. This root has been shown to increase attention span and memory, increase sexual stimulation, add strength and display anti-toxic action, which increases anti-tumor activity by supporting the body's ability to resist harmful toxins. Especially beneficial for seniors, it regulates the central nervous system and helps to keep brain chemistry balanced.

Rhododendron caucasicum. In the Republic of Georgia, formerly part of the Soviet Union, it is not unusual for people to live beyond 100 years of age as active members of society. When Russians marry, they propose a toast to the bride and groom, gifting them Georgian longevity. What is their secret? For over 2,000 years Georgians have consumed herbal Alpine Tea as a daily ritual, along with grain kefir, containing eleven different probiotics. In addition, the water they drink is full of glacial minerals. It has been theorized that their long lives may be attributed to regular consumption of this traditional yogurt (kefir), and flavonoids-rich foods such as wine and honey along with their Alpine Tea.

       The last verifiable statistics from the Republic of Georgia show that there are almost 23,000 Georgians over the age of 100, based on a population of only 3.2 million people. One of the key reasons for their longevity is Rhododendron Caucasicum, the ingredient in Alpine Tea. Grown at the 10 to 13,000 foot elevations in the Caucasian Mountains, Rhododendron Caucasicum (also known as snow rose) contains polyphenolics, including flavonoids and proanthocyanidins. Thirty years of research indicate that the phenylpropanoids in Rhododendron improve physical abilities, increase activity of the cardiovascular system, and increase blood supply to the muscles, and especially to the brain. Rhododendron Caucasicum increases resistance of the brain to imbalances due to chemical, physical and biological reasons. It also is an anti-bacterial, while allowing the good probiotics to thrive. It acts as a detoxicant, is highly P-Vitamin active, protecting against capillary fragility, and is an excellent free-radical scavenger. Studies have demonstrated that Rhododendron Caucasicum inhibits or abolishes the activity of the enzyme Hyaluronidase, known to be an initiator of colon cancer.

Clinical research has been ongoing as to the medicinal uses of this alpine plant. Professor Dimitry M. Rossiyski, M.D. Meritorious Science Worker at the U.S.S.R. Medical Academy of Science, conducted a double-blind placebo study on seventy test subjects diagnosed with circulatory insufficiency and atherosclerosis, some with high blood pressure and evidence of past heart attacks. A 30mg/day dose of Rhododendron extract over a 15 day period, resulted in the subjects experiencing a lowered blood pressure, improvement in coronary circulation, decrease of serum cholesterol and elimination of pain in the chest area.

Subsequent studies at the First Central Moscow Hospital, showed similar results on heart patients suffering from hardening of the arteries. Doctors Avraamova and Galperin performed clinical studies at the Moscow State Hospital on 24 males and 36 females, ages 18-65, diagnosed with Mitral Valve insufficiency (prolapsed). Improvements were obvious in the patients taking Rhodendron extract, over those who did not receive it. The average heart beats in those receiving the extract were lowered from 90 to 70 beats per minute, and systolic blood pressure was lowered from 177 to 160 mm Hg. (Rossiysky 1954).

Again, studies at the First Central Moscow Hospital revealed that when 50 mgs. of Rhododendron Caucasicum, diluted in water, was given to 170 volunteers suffering from severe gout, the average discharge of uric acid increased 55-60 per cent and pain was relieved in a few hours. The Georgian Academy of Sciences gave 50 to 100 mgs. per day of the snow rose to 114 patients hospitalized for depression. The results showed a marked decrease in depressive symptoms in 93 of the patients. Similar results were achieved by the Moscow State Hospital study, indicating improvement of 162 patients with severe depression.

Rhododendron is also highly antibacterial, perhaps due to the presence of the well-known antibacterial compounds Chlorogenic and caffeic acids, that are known to exist in this plant. Tests conclude that it is more effective than either Grape Seed or Pine Bark as an antibacterial proanthocyanidin. In a 24 hour test of 12,000 Staphylococcus aureus bacteria thriving in solution, all were totally eliminated by Rhododendron, but 300 colonies were still surviving in the Grape Seed petri dish, and 370 in the Pine Bark solution. Rhododendron is more synergistic to the human body, because the extraction process is not accomplished using organic solvents, which are a source of the very free radicals the proanthocyanidins are trying to eliminate. This method is customary in extraction of Grape Seed or Pine Bark.

Rhododendron Caucasicum is a unique plant among all other species of Rhododendrons, and considered safe for human consumption. It is reported that some Rhododendrons, mainly flowers, contain Grayanotoxins which are not soluble in water and can be harmful. Therefore, do not just go out to your garden and harvest your backyard Rhododendron. The snow rose has been used in foreign hospitals to treat heart disease, arthritis, gout, high cholesterol, blood pressure problems, depression, neuroses and psychoses and concentration problems. Along with a strong regime of probiotic supplementation, and maintaining a healthy mineral balance in your body, taking Rhododendron Caucasicum may give your body the tools it needs to achieve the level of longevity enjoyed by the elder Georgians.

SKIN

Young fresh skin is no longer an illusion. From time immemorial, beauty and a youthful appearance have moved hearts. Today skin care, and particularly facial care, is an important element of the conscious experience of well being, personality, attractiveness, and individuality. Skin problems manifest because there is something happening inside the body that reflects in our outward appearance. Treating these problems may help, but it is imperative that we discover the cause of the wrinkle or blemish in order to effect a permanent cure.

Beautiful skin is more than skin deep. The skin is the largest organ of nourishment and elimination, with the acid mantle, or covering of the skin, inhibiting the growth of disease-causing bacteria. Skin problems are one of the surest signs of poor nutrition, and improved nutrition is quickly mirrored by skin health. Some of the causes of skin problems are emotional stress, poor diet of refined foods and sugar, too many saturated fats, caffeine overload, food allergies, liver malfunction, poor digestion and assimilation, irritating cosmetics, essential fatty acid depletion, synthetic fiber clothing, PMS and menopausal changes.

Beginning at the age of thirty, there is a reduction of elastin and collagen (fibrous protein) production in the connective tissue where the elastic and collagen fibers are found. The skin enzyme, elastase, attacks the elastic fibers and destroys the elastic, therefore your skin loses its tone. The contour of your skin, wrinkles and lines are determined by many factors, including moisture and the relative health of collagen. Aging of the skin occurs when collagen becomes hard and crosslinked with neighboring collagen fibers. The cause of the crosslinking is oxidation, or free-radical formation. Free radicals attack cell membranes, genetic cell material, and the collagen and elastin proteins causing wrinkles, sagging contours, sallow complexion and skin cancer. Some of the causes of free radical damage are smog and environment pollutants, too much sunlight (UVA and UVB), stress, poor diet, liver exhaustion, and skin dehydration caused by estrogen depletion.

Silica is a combination of silicon and oxygen. Found in unprocessed oats, barley, millet, wheat and potatoes, it plays a strong role in maintaining health of our skin, hair and nails. It is needed to create collagen which cannot be formed without abundant levels of silica and vitamin C. The body's levels of silica decline as we age resulting in the signs of aging that appear in our skin, therefore it may be necessary to supplement our diets with silica. It is especially useful as a treatment for thinning hair, dry skin, brittle nails and dandruff.

The newly discovered algae extract, aosain, protects and strengthens the connective tissue, and counteracts the loss of elasticity in the skin. Aosain is obtained from the Aosa Algae, which is so elastic it endures the stormy seas of Brittany without being smashed on the rocks. Applied topically, this protective mechanism of the algae extract, when transported into the deeper layers of the epidermis, retards the damaging effects of the elastase enzyme, and so counteracts the natural reduction of elastin. Active almond protein also can stimulate the production of collagen and elastin to prevent loss and firm tone. Vitamin A and E stimulate cell regeneration and support skin regeneration. Vitamin E can also protect against free radical damage.

The skin's moisture content begins to diminish early in life. After age 30, up to 25 percent is lost, and by age 40, as much as 50 percent is lost. Wrinkles and sagging skin are evidence of skin dehydration. A billion dollar industry has developed to provide products that will keep moisture in skin as it ages. Unfortunately, most of these creams, lotions, etc. are plastered on the skin to try and keep moisture in. If the skin is moisture deficient, wouldn't it be smarter to add moisture, as well as try to retain moisture? Drinking our eight glasses of purified water a day can make a big difference in rehydrating the skin. Also, eliminate dehydrants such as caffeine, from your diet.

We can also spray our face with a substance containing humectants, a substance that causes a cactus to draw moisture out of the desert air. Our bodies also produce their own humectants, specifically, NaPCA. This natural moisturizer can be produced synthetically in a laboratory. Both types are derived from glutamic acid, one of the non-essential amino acids occurring in humans. NaPCA, present on our skin surface, may be a direct cause of glowing natural beauty, while its decline brings on the deep furrows and inelasticity of age. The skin has the ability to hold moisture, and as the level of NaPCA decreases with age, the moisture content of the skin begins to drop as well. NaPCA is a water soluble substance, light enough for any skin to use and available commercially as a body spray, and within skin care products.

Herbs, when combined with crystalloid trace minerals (electrolytes), can be a nourishing complement in a moisturizing skin spray. These nutrients penetrate to the deepest layers of the skin, carrying oxygen molecules across the cell wall. Electrolytes enhance tissue oxygenation, aiding the reduction of free radical formation, and can be a major factor in slowing down our skin's aging process! Crystalloid trace minerals, which give 100 percent solubility, penetrate the epidermal barrier, rejuvenating cell function of the deepest layer where skin is made. The minerals also capture and stabilize free-radicals before they damage and wrinkle skin. Wheat germ protein, macadamia nut oil and moisture-retaining hyaluronic acid can smooth fine lines caused by dry skin.

Combinations of various healing herbs such as aloe vera, horsetail (silica), chamomile, comfrey, and burdock root, when bonded with electrolytes, readily enters the bloodstream and penetrates the cells of the body. This initiates a healing response that benefits the entire organism, similar to a full symphony orchestra coming into play. Electrolytes are a trans-dermal nutrient healer and an important aid to skin rejuvenation. Good skin hydration is one of the most important aspects of attaining and maintaining youthful skin.

Keeping your immune system in tip-top shape will result in a healthy, young outer appearance. In addition to nutrients mentioned in other chapters, sea vegetables, taken internally, play a large part in the health of your skin. Seaweed has a composition so close to human plasma that it can help balance the cells of the body. Seaweed, kelp, and red marine algae, help nourish and hydrate aging skin when used both topically and internally. Calcium and magnesium in seaweed drain fluid out of tissues, helping to fight water retention and reduce cellulite. Red marine algae helps the cells to grow rapidly, improve skin firmness and elasticity, and results in smoother, less lined skin. Using these natural plants from the water can quickly control or eliminate fingernail fungus, athlete's foot or other fungal infections of the skin.

As we said before, aging skin is a reflection of a toxic body. Minerals will help your hair growth, reduce gray, keep your hair and fingernails strong and create an energy glow in your face. As a basic tool for the immune system, minerals strengthen the entire body. You face reflects your internal condition. Watch it get younger looking as your body gets healthier. For more detailed information on natural skin care treatments, please read our booklet, *The Guide To All Natural Anti-Aging Skin Care.*

HORMONAL IMBALANCES.

Fifty is a milestone for both men and women because their bodily changes are becoming obvious, not normally for the better. Aches, pains and threat of debilitating disease become a closer reality. It is our belief that both men and women are affected by hormonal changes and although men don't get hot flashes, they can be affected by the other conditions described in this chapter.

Estrogen and progesterone supplementation is not fully understood by menopausal people who may be abusing their bodies with these creams and pills. When estrogen and progesterone levels decrease, the slack is picked up by the adrenal glands. If our bodies are stressed, our adrenals become exhausted and are unable to produce the needed hormones. Androgens (specifically andros-tenedione, an adrenal hormone) can be converted to estrogen in both men and women. Men's estrogen level production goes up as their testosterone levels decrease. In post-menopausal women, the conversion of androgens and progesterone to estrogen can occur if thyroid function is inadequate. Adrenal glands are the main source of estrogen when the ovaries slow their production during menopause. If the adrenals are stressed and functioning poorly before menopause, they cannot produce the needed estrogen when menopause begins.

Estrogen refers to a class of hormones with estrus activity (prepares the woman for pregnancy). These include estradiol and estrone. Both are implicated in stimulating abnormal cell growth when occurring in higher than normal amounts in the body. Estrogens also include estriol, which is know to be cancer inhibiting. If you find low levels of estrogen (saliva tests can more accurately determine this than blood tests), it is best to supplement with natural estrogens. An excellent food that has estrogenic qualities is soy. As mentioned elsewhere in this book, soy is extremely beneficial when taken in fermented form, such as foods that include tempe and miso. Sprouted soy is also available in powdered or capsule supplements. It comes with no side effects, and because it is a food assimilated by the body, it does not contribute to an over-estrogen condition. Soy contains weak estrogens, or isoflavones, which compete with the full strength estrogenic hormones for access to the cells. Isoflavones bind with cell receptors that would normally attract the body's own estrogen, but the growth signal they deliver is only $1/1000^{th}$ as strong, thus reducing the risk of cancer from excess estrogen.

Excess estrogen from estrogen replacement therapy (ERT) may increase the growth of existing cancers, unless it balanced by progesterone. It can create other side effects as well such as increased risk of pituitary, uterine and breast cancers, liver dysfunction, gall bladder attacks, the likelihood of breast fibrocysts, uterine fibroids, water retention, and weight gain. Estrogen replacement therapy must always include a healthy ratio of progesterone to estrogen of ten to one.

You may be getting excess estrogen without even taking a supplement. Many chemicals (called xeno-estrogens) mimic estrogen in the body. These include chlorine, pesticides and petroleum byproducts, and ingredients in spermicides contained in condom and vaginal gels. Excess estrogen is also associated with heart problems, stroke and hypoxia (lack of oxygen). Women who have ratios of less than five progesterone to one estrogen, are prone to cyclic seizures, excessive bleeding, fibrocystic breast disease, and ovarian cysts. It also promotes thyroid deficiencies because it inhibits thyroid secretion. This results in symptoms such as headaches, frequent infections, insomnia, fatigue, depression, constipation, cancer and squamous metaplasia in prostate cells, a precancerous condition, to name a few. Men can experience an over-estrogen condition, whereby they develop higher voices and breast fat as they age.

Supplementing with natural progesterone can help many over-estrogen conditions. Progesterone is the precursor of both estrogen and testosterone, and adrenocortical hormones that regulate sugar and electrolyte balance and blood pressure. Progesterone deficiency can seriously affect bones and is a concern in the development of osteoporosis. Many doctors prescribe estrogen replacement to ward off osteoporosis. In fact, the extra estrogen will unbalance the progesterone and may possibly accelerate osteoporosis. Progesterone stimulates osteoblast-mediated new bone formation, which results in the growth of new bone tissue and a reversal of the osteoporosis at any age.

When using natural progesterone, you must ask questions of the manufacturer. Natural progesterone actually stimulates its own synthesis in the body. Natural progesterone is not the same as synthetic progestins which have side effects such as depression, acne, and weight gain. Synthetic progestins may be carcinogenic, and inhibit the production of your own natural progesterone. Semi-synthetic progesterone, if used as an isolate, is known as Progesterone U.S.P. Although it is extracted from wild yams, it may not include some of the plant's natural enzymes, peptides or other phytosterols having been destroyed in the extraction process. These are important phytochemicals the body needs to nurture itself.

Semi-synthetic progesterone may be quite effective in reducing menopausal symptoms at the onset, but it may have undesirable long-term side effects. Even a small dosage of 25mg/day can block pathways in the endocrine system, raising cholesterol levels and requiring stronger and stronger dosages to work, as it will eventually desensitize receptor sites.

Progesterone replacement is best accomplished by using a product containing Progesterone U.S.P., along with wild yam (Dioscorea). Organically grown Mexican wild yam whole plant extract, has a modulating or balancing effect on how the body utilizes the progesterone isolate. The resultant product is nearly identical to the progesterone that the body produces. The method of extraction must be one that leaves all the nutrients intact. James

Jamieson, pharmacologist, is currently working with over 110 species of wild yams. He states, "You have to be careful not to disturb the delicate synergism and balance as each phytogen, peptide, enzyme, co-enzyme as well as other co-factors because they all have different and remarkable actions and activities in the body."

Synthetic, semi-synthetic and many natural progesterones do not respect mother nature's wisdom, and will provide only that substance that gets immediate results. Also, many wild yam creams or tinctures can be hazardous to your health, because they contain pesticides, whose residue will mimic pseudoestrogens and definitely destroy the endocrine balance. Be sure that your wild yam supplement of choice is organic and has all its natural nutrients intact. A simple natural approach to reducing an over-estrogen condition is by simply adding flax to your diet. As mentioned in the chapter on fats, you can consume flax oil, pulverized flax meal or you can grind your own flax seed (organic, of course).

Herbal treatments for hormonal imbalance have been used for centuries. Herbs, being natural, seem to create a synergistic harmony with the body and therefore may be a more natural choice in reducing symptoms. Maca (Peruvian ginseng) has been used by the Incas for both nutritional and medicinal purposes. It enhances female fertility, treats male impotence, and helps with menstrual irregularities and has been used to treat female hormonal imbalances, including menopause. It is a nutritional powerhouse that is especially rich in iodine, amino acids, complex carbohydrates and essential minerals such as iron, zinc, phosphorus, calcium and magnesium. Maca also contains various vitamins such as B1, B2, B12, C and E.

Black cohosh is used in female gland toning compounds for PMS, menstrual problems and menopausal symptoms. It helps increase fertility by regulating hormone production, especially after discontinuing the birth control pill. Chaste Tree berry assists in normalizing a woman's sex drive, stimulating production of progesterone by balancing abnormally high estrogen levels. It helps for depression, headaches, premenstrual acne, breast tenderness, cramps and bloating.

Dendrobium leaf (Chinese Herb) nourishes sensitive vaginal tissue by increasing body fluids. Combined with Licorice, it re-balances the hormonal levels. Dong Quai restores a woman to hormone harmony. It is often called the female ginseng, because it acts as an adaptogen (regulator) to maintain a woman's proper deep body balance. This herb may alleviate hot flashes and vaginal atrophy during menopause. Dong Quai has been called the queen of all female herbs. Ginseng (Siberian) help's restore a woman's body balance, both physically and biochemically. It assists in preserving the health of female organs, especially in cases where natural estrogen is absent, such as following a hysterectomy. It also prevents vaginal atrophy, modulates hormone release, improves fertility, boosts energy and relieves the irritability of pre-menopause and menopause.

Licorice contains traces of phytoestrogen sterols similar to those produced by the adrenal glands. It increases longevity and improves erotic arousal and stamina. Licorice has a normalizing effect on the body for fluid retention, breast tenderness, abdominal bloating, mood swings as well as depression. Sarsaparilla is an excellent hormone balancing herb for both men and women. It contains the male hormone testosterone, progesterone and cortin which stimulate the action of estrogen in females.

As our levels of testosterone decrease, it may be necessary to give them a boost. Research has shown that ginseng contains plant testosterone, and is the only known herb that can stimulate production of testosterone in the body. Tribulus terrestis (puncture vine) is most commonly found in the Indian subcontinent and Africa. It has been used since ancient times in India as a treatment for sexual dysfunction. The most common cross-cultural use of the tribulus terrestis herb has been in the treatment of infertility in women, impotence in men and for increasing libido of both sexes. Tribulus appears to raise the testosterone production in men via the activation of leutinizing hormone (LH) secretion from the pituitary gland. The benefit of tribulus on the endocrine system and hormone production is believed to be largely due to its action in the liver. It acts as a liver tonic, improving the emulsification of fats to essential fatty acids, which along with cholesterol, is used by the liver to manufacture hormones.

We asked Dr. Linda Rector Page to comment on some of the other popular hormone therapies. The information is extracted from her Natural Healing Report, September 1998. ANDRO (Androstenedione) is a by-product of DHEA, with the commercial product being synthesized from the seeds of the Scotch Pine tree. It is a direct precursor to testosterone and has a powerful effect on hormone health and balance. In some studies, for short periods of time it actually increased the body's testosterone supply up to three times the normal level.

This drug is most popular among bodybuilders and athletes who want to increase muscle mass. It is best used by men and women who have a proven testosterone deficiency. It is also used to help maintain bone density and offset osteoporosis. For people with sports injuries, it has the benefit of being able to boost metabolism and stimulate the repair of damaged tissue. The negative side of ANDRO is that little is known about its long-term side effects. What is known is that it can boost testosterone levels too much and too fast, causing excess testosterone as well as aggressive behavior and acne.

Too much testosterone may convert into estrogen-causing breast enlargement (in men too) or water retention. Women can start to grow facial whiskers, chest hair or find their voice deepens. Teens should be wary, as it may stunt growth and cause permanent damage to the heart and liver. As with any hormone replacement, the body may perceive abnormal amounts of this synthetic hormone, and shut down its normal production after long term use.

Natural alternatives to ANDRO could be the herb ginseng, which has a rejuvenating, tonic action on the male body, and has a history of being safe. CoQ10, an enzyme supplement, can improve physical performance and increase cellular energy safely. Also, a highly concentrated extract from the nettle root provides a unique mechanism for increasing levels of free testosterone. Nettle root binds to the hormone that controls levels of free testosterone, known as sex hormone binding globulin (SHBG), in place of testosterone. This reduces SHBG's binding of free testosterone.

Pregnenolone (called PREG) is a steroid hormone made primarily in the adrenal glands from cholesterol and is the precursor to DHEA and progesterone in the body. PREG supplements are synthesized in the laboratory from wild yam diosgenin which leads people to believe it is safe. PREG does produce a feeling of well-being, increases energy levels, enhance visual and auditory perception and leads to better awareness and alertness. The downside is that it induces central nervous system excitability and can cause insomnia, or shallow sleep. High dosages can cause irritability, anger or anxiety, and doses over 25 mg. may cause headaches. No serious adverse effects have been documented, but few studies have been performed; therefore, not much is really known about potential long-term hazards. Natural alternatives are gotu kola, a ginseng-like adaptogen herb, which is an excellent nervous system restorative that can increase mental energy, promote a sense of well-being and heighten sensations without safety risks. For mental clarity you may add American ginseng and ginkgo biloba.

DHEA (dehydroepiandrosterone) is the most abundant steroid hormone made by your adrenal glands. Synthetic DHEA is synthesized in laboratories from the steroidal saponin (diosgenin), a steroid-like component of the wild yam plant. It appears to enhance a sense of well-being and improve libido, especially in those people with low testosterone. DHEA reduces chronic pain, is helpful in increasing bone density, reduce the risk of inappropriate blood clotting.

The downside of DHEA is that it can induce adult acne, perspiration, facial hair growth and head hair loss. It also may cause irritability, insomnia and mood swings, as well as confusion, headaches and liver damage. It is not recommended for people with ovarian, thyroid or adrenal tumors. Though DHEA is promoted as an anti-aging hormone, studies with mice suggest it may actually shorten life spans. Health experts are concerned that using DHEA for a year or more at high dosages (50 mg or more/day) may be linked to breast, ovary and prostate tumor growth.

Dr. Page mentions that breakthrough technology may increase your body's own production of DHEA. Dr. C. Norman Shealy, M.D., Ph.D. uses a subtle electrical nerve stimulator and incorporates synthesized progesterone cream to stimulate 12 acupuncture points that boost your own DHEA production naturally. Also, a combination of royal jelly and Chinese red ginseng is a powerful hormone stimulant and aphrodisiac for women, without the side effects of masculinization or health risks of DHEA.

Melatonin is nature's sleeping ill. Melatonin supplements are pharmaceutically synthesized from chemically altered serotonin. Natural melatonin is actually available too, but some products are derived from the pineal gland of cattle that may contain contaminants (antibiotic residue or other drugs.) Melatonin is safe if used wisely for specific purpose. It does help reduce the effects of jet lag when traveling, and it can be used for chronic insomnia. It also has been known to decrease the size of the prostate gland (because a melatonin deficiency allows it to grow). It can also help with low-tryptophan diseases such as anorexia, hypertension and some types of depression.

Used daily, melatonin can actually worsen sleep. In a Consumer Report's poll of 400 people with sleep problems, 50% said melatonin did not help and only 25% thought it was beneficial.

Side effects can show up as causing nightmares, nausea, stomach cramps, and it can even shrink male gonads and decrease sex drive. A study from Singapore revealed that long-term users may experience an eventual shutdown of their body's own production of melatonin. For natural alternatives, seek out tryptophan rich foods such as chicken, turkey, pumpkin seeds and cottage cheese. Nervine sedative herbs like valerian and skullcap enhance your quality of sleep and your dreams. There are melatonin alternatives for jet lag, including homeopathic preparations, and using a strong full spectrum light to reset your body clock.

As we have mentioned in this chapter, the choice for hormone therapy is up to you. Each person reacts differently and there is no one magic pill for everyone. We strongly advise that you do not take hormone replacement supplementation lightly. You should determine your levels and your deficiencies before indiscriminately popping a hormone pill. It is best to talk to your physician or an alternative health practitioner prior to undertaking a hormone replacement program. There are many occasions where natural hormone supplementation may be extremely beneficial, but you should not make that decision without proper testing.

Recommended reading:

•*Hormone Heresy*, by Sherrill Sellman
Get Well International Publishing
•*Dr. Linda Page's Natural Healing Report*, Linda Page, N.D., Ph.D.
Weiss Research Inc., (800) 408-0081

DIS-EASES OF AGING

Remedies excerpted from some of the following sources:
Healing Nutrients by Dr. P. Quillan; The Biochemic Handbook by J.B. Chapman, MD
and Edward L. Perry, MD; Traditional Home & Herbal Remedies by Jan De Vries,
Naturopathic Handbook of Herbal Formulas, information on flower remedies supplied
by Natural Labs, Homeopathic remedies supplied by Bioforce and Homeopathic Works,
herbal suggestions by Linda Rector Page's Healthy Healing book, and herbs used in
Traditional Chinese Medicine by the Connecticut Institute of Herbal Studies,

—Note: Compounded means combined, (in listing of herbal remedies). The symbol *
next to an herb name in the text refers to Chinese herbs.

AGE SPOTS.
These are nothing more than external signs of harmful waste accumulation that cannot find an easy way out of the body. This cellular debris lodges in the skin and shows up as discoloration. Lipofuscin is the age-related skin pigment that oxidizes to actually appear as the brown age spot. Free radical damage caused by environmental pollution, over exposure to the sun, stress, and poor diet can set the stage for a break down in the toxin elimination process. Liver malfunction, smoking, broken capillaries, weak vein walls, and poor food assimilation are also contributing factors. The best way to reduce these age spots is to clean house. Go on a good detoxification program, especially one designed to clean the liver. Supplements like royal jelly, shark liver oil, essential fatty acids and vitamin C can assist in the cleansing process. Herbal helpers can include dandelion, *ginseng, gotu kola, licorice and sarsaparilla. bilberry also helps slow the aging process because it is an anti-oxidant, stabilizes connecting tissue and strengthens blood vessels.

As we mentioned in a previous chapter when explaining micronutrients from the sun, the primary energy compound converted from sunlight is known as ATP. Harvested plants provide our cells with energized food so they can make this ATP, which nourishes our cells and slows the aging process. This new process becomes the facilitator to recharge our cellular structure. The proteins, when charged, reject free radicals. This results in less damage to our internal organs and prevents cells from dying (anti-aging). With less cells dying, less debris is floating around our system and lodging under our skin as age spots. The solution that provides this ATP is made from concentrated organic fruit juices, honey and teas through a solar distillation process that changes the sun's power into chemical energy that can be used by the body.

ARTHRITIS.
Considered by some to be an inevitable part of aging, arthritis is thought to be caused by a toxic body trying to rid itself of waste. When salts combine with other wastes, they precipitate out of the blood and lymph fluids, forming abrasive deposits. These end up in the joints causing bursitis and arthritis which may also be caused or aggravated by the demineralization of the bones necessary to service our mineral deficient bodies.

Since most of our foods and water are lacking minerals, it is necessary to replace them with a crystalloid electrolyte supplement. Arthritis may be caused by cortisone drugs which, if taken over a long period of time, tend to affect the solidity of bone. In order to avoid an arthritic condition, it is very important to maintain a toxic-free lifestyle, thereby freeing the body from its arduous task of removing these toxins.

In the chapter, *Essential Fatty Acids*, we discussed the use of GLA (Gamma Linolenic Acid) from borage, Evening Primrose & black currant oils. Applications of these oils as it applies to rheumatoid arthritis has shown to be effective in reducing inflammation and joint tenderness. All GLA oils have the ability to effect these results, although larger dosages are required of Evening Primrose and black currant oils than borage oil.

Cleansing and supporting the immune system will help reduce the effects of arthritis in the long run. For relatively immediate relief, drink black cherry juice (best to use the concentrate diluted in water or juice), and use royal jelly (from worker bees). Herbal remedies containing nettles, red cover, compounded juniper berry, compounded yucca/burdock, garlic, seaweed and nutritional yeast are great alternatives to a pain pill. Cayenne pepper capsules can bring blood to the joints and muscles to keep them warm and flexible, especially if you are living a sedentary lifestyle.

A home treatment could include the following procedure: In the morning, drink a half a glass of raw potato juice on an empty stomach (or dilute with warm water). Eat organic foods. An hour before lunch, eat 2-3 Juniper berries. After lunch, eat 2-4 whole mustard seeds. During the day, drink the water organic potatoes were boiled in. Cabbage juice and black cherry juice also have been known to reduce the symptoms of arthritis. Taking extra calcium and magnesium, and drinking goat's milk may improve the condition.

Herbs that can help are Una de gato, compounded red clover, nettles, compounded yucca/burdock, and compounded devil's claw/chaparral. Instead of eating juniper berries, take them in a liquid herbal tincture. There are specific herbal agents that influence certain kinds of arthritis, and you should consult an herbologist for these.

If you have bearing-down type of pain in the lower back combined with a tired feeling, you may consider a homeopathic tissue salt, Calc. Fluor. (Calcium Fluoride) which helps to preserve the power of elastic tissue to contract. Mag. Phos. (Magnesium Phosphate) is also good for steady sharp neuralgic pains in the back, as it is an anti-spasmodic. MSM, Methyl Sulfonyl Methane is a naturally occurring, organic form of the element sulfur, which the body uses to create new healthy cells. As a supplement, it can be effective against arthritis. Garlic, nutritional yeast and kelp can help pain, and cayenne pepper can help the joints to be more flexible. For lower back pain, use *Wen Yang (Modified Eucommia and Rehmannia formula).

Osteoarthritis. Also called degenerative joint disease, osteoarthritis is one of the oldest and most common types of arthritis. It is characterized by the breakdown of the joint's cartilage, which causes the surface bone to rub against the opposing bone, resulting in pain and loss of movement. This disease normally affects the hands, knees hips, feet and back, but can also cause problems in the blood vessels, kidneys, skin, eyes and brain. Contributing factors are obesity, joint inflammation, chronic infections and years of repetitive use.

One theory about the overall cause of arthritis has to do with the abnormal release of the enzyme Hyaluronidase from the cartilage cells. This enzyme is known in medical research literature to play a crucial role in the activation of procarcinogens (PCG), which initiate cancerous activity in the colon. Factors that influence this enzyme are diet, pH, and microbial ecology in the colon (bad vs. good bacteria). Hyaluronidase breaks down the Hyaluronic acid that is an essential constituent in collagen. An herbal extract from the Rhododenron caucasicum plant has shown ability to inhibit the activity of Hyaluronidase, thereby possibly acting to protect the body from osteoarthritis.

Supplements such as glucosamine, which rehydrates cartilage, giving it greater cushioning power, may actually lead to the rebuilding of cartilage with long-term usage. Cartilage is a mass of collagen fibers embedded in a glue-like ground substance called chondrin which is made up of about 20% protein and 80% carbohydrates. Special cells (chondrocytes) within the cartilage synthesize both the collagen fibers and the chondrin matrix which holds them. Chondroitin sulfate and glucosamine are used by the chondrocytes in the manufacture of chondrin.

Glucosamine and chondroitin sulfate play an important part, and can be found in supplement form as well as in Velvet antler, traditionally taken as a tonic for stress and fatigue. Scientific literature from Russia, China and Korea reports the anti-inflammatory properties of antler velvet extracts, which could explain the traditional usage as a tonic for arthritis and similar inflammatory conditions. Neither chondroitin sulfate nor glucosamine supply the amino acid building blocks for the proteins in collagen; therefore, they cannot be utilized to rebuild the *entire* structure of cartilage. They do not contribute to the manufacture of a major component of cartilage, the collagen fibers. Hydrolyzed bovine collagen, produced in Germany after extensive clinical research, has demonstrated ability to rebuild cartilage. With the support of trace minerals, the enzymes in the chondrocytes are fueled so the reconstruction can take place. Since these chondrocytes never lose their ability to build cartilage, even after a dormant period, bathing them in essential nutrients can bring back their productivity.

BALDNESS OR THINNING HAIR.
This is a main concern of the aging population. Balding is not necessarily genetic or permanent, and sometimes may be related to oxygen starvation of the cells in the scalp. It can be precipitated by the over consumption of certain dietary fats, such as hydrogenated oil and unfermented soybean products.

In a test it was found that sheep that ate a diet of raw soybean plants experienced a loss of hair. It seems the unfermented soybean has a biochemical component, phyto-hemagglutinin, that may act as a glue in the blood, contributing to hair loss. Fat-laden blood goes directly to the head, where the soy oil causes the red blood cells to stick together and plug the blood capillaries. This will reduce the oxygen to the scalp and the hair follicles, and literally smother the scalp. Gray hair can be caused by this condition, and also by vitamin deficiencies. De-toxing and rebuilding the immune system may clear out these clogged areas and provide a healthy environment for new hair growth. Eliminating trans-fatty acids (hydrogenated oils) and unfermented soy products from your diet, may help you guard against baldness.

Depending on what has caused the condition, these treatments may work. Rinse the scalp with vinegar and Sage tea. Take 40 drops of liquid Red Clover tops daily and 30-60 mg. of zinc. You can also rub aloe vera in the scalp. Another treatment is to drink tea on a daily basis, made from stinging nettle, walnut leaves and elder leaves. Silica is necessary for hair growth. Aging depletes this essential element and if replenished may correct a thinning hair condition. Biochemic cell salt treatment can include Kali. Sulph. (Potassium Sulphate) for falling-out hair and bald spots, as well as Nat. Mur. (Sodium Chloride). Bee pollen has worked for some people, who not only had their hair grow back, but it turned gray back to color. To help restore hair color use *Shou Wu Chih (Radix Polygoni Multifori).

BLOOD CLOTS AND CIRCULATION.
Another fear of aging people is blood clots, because they can break loose and go to places in the body that threaten life's functions. The body has the unique ability to determine when blood should clot and when it should stay fluid. Blood platelets normally are disc-like; however, when the body requires clotting for wound repair, these same discs grow projecting arms that interlock to hold them together. This process is facilitated by, and also dependent upon, a host of molecular and cellular activities. The danger comes when these clots travel in the bloodstream to places such as the heart or brain. Aged garlic extract, and its active compounds, are potent inhibitors of those substances that hold the clots together, and thus is an effective blood thinner with virtually no side effects.

One of the most powerful natural circulatory stimulants, Cayenne red pepper gets the blood moving to everywhere it is needed. In his book, *Left for Dead*, author Dick Quinn chronicles the use of the hot herb for circulatory problems, ranging from heart disease and high blood pressure, to ulcers and impotence. The power of cayenne is measured in heat units. The

108

culinary spice is only about 2,000 heat units whereas supplemental cayenne comes in 40-120,000 heat unit products. In his book, Dick Quinn suggests 2 capsules, 3 times a day to boost circulation.

Ginkgo biloba is an important herb for strength, vitality, mental alertness, and to improve the blood flow in small veins. It is extremely beneficial in the treatment of erectile dysfunction caused by lack of blood flow to the penis. Ginkgo also is a primary brain and mental energy stimulant, enhancing cerebral circulation. The herb, damiana has been found to contain several alkaloids that directly stimulate the nerves, increase circulation, and have muscle-relaxant properties.

CANCER.

This is a topic all in itself. We will not go into length on this subject, other than to provide information on a few treatments that we know are used to prevent cancer. We will, however, touch on the fact that low progesterone levels have been related to increased incidences of breast and uterine cancer. Evidence suggests that breast cancer occurs most often at the stage of life when estrogen is dominant for a full month in a woman's cycle, and progesterone is missing or minimal (unbalanced menstrual cycles). The American Journal of Epidemiology in 1981 published forty years of research by John Hopkins Private Obstetrics and Gynecology clinic, revealing that the occurrence of breast cancer was 5.4 times greater in the women who had low levels of progesterone. This is extremely important when we consider many doctors prescribe estrogen replacement therapy to guard against cancer, when in fact, it is just the reverse. Progesterone replacement therapy should be given to offset the over-estrogen condition.

Foods are getting good press lately as cancer fighters. Aged garlic extract and its constituents S-allyl cysteine, allixin and diallyl sulfide, have been shown to inhibit breast cancer, bladder cancer, melanoma cells, skin, liver, lung and colon cancer. A prime carcinogen, aflatoxin B. (AFB), is linked with liver cancer and is produced by Aspergillus mold in contaminated peanuts, rice, cereal grains, corn, beans and sweet potatoes. AFB in its natural unmetabolized form is actually not damaging to the body. Once it enters the body, the enzyme system metabolizes and chemically reacts to it. Some of the products of this metabolism can bind to DNA and cause trouble. Our bodies do produce enzymes that can make AFB less toxic and excrete it from our body. Aged garlic can help by inhibiting the AFB from binding with the DNA and hastening the excretion of this toxin from the body, thus giving us protection from this risk of liver cancer.

Tocotrienols are close cousins to tocopherols (vitamin E) as a powerful antioxidant. They have anticancer activity without any side effects, directly inhibiting the growth of human breast cancer cells by 50%. Tocotrienols are found along with vitamin E in grains such as barley, soybeans, rice, amaranth and others. They differ from tocopherols by a specific molecular structure which, although minute, does relate to a large difference in effectiveness. They also have been shown to fight against melanoma type cancers. True vegetarians who consume large quantities of tocotrienol-containing foods may achieve this type of antioxidant success, but for the rest of us, supplementation with a product containing concentrations of tocotrienols may be necessary.

Antioxidants such as the polyphenols in green tea (20 times more effective than vitamin E) and the lycopene in tomatoes, help neutralize the free radical that can damage a cell's DNA and limit its cancer fighting ability. Broccoli, cauliflower and other cruciferous vegetables boost production of phase II enzymes necessary to cart off cancer-causing chemical residue. Flax and its abundance of omega-3 essential fatty acid, thwart tumor growth by pushing harmful saturated fats out of our cells. Soy, rosemary, carrots and grapes also contain a compound known as Cox-2 inhibitors. These impede the growth of new blood vessels, and when tested on cancer cells, actually reduced the growth factor that caused cancer cells to proliferate. With researchers estimating that diets filled with fruits and vegetables could eventually reduce cancer incidence by 30-40%, everyone should consider watching their food choices.

Essiac, an herbal tea formula of the Ojibway Indians was made famous for treating cancer by Rene Caisse. The formula consists of sheep sorrel, burdock root, turkey rhubarb and slippery elm bark. There is universal agreement among natural healers, both past and present, that detoxifiying your body is the key to healing and strengthening the immune system. Essiac has proven itself to be effective not only against cancer, but against a multiplicity of other diseases including MS, CFS, Arthritis and Parkinson's disease.

EYE DISORDERS:

Cataracts. These are opaque clusters of dead protein cells in the crystalline lens of the eye that reflect light, rather than letting it pass through to the retina. The result is a gradual and painless loss of vision. Cataracts are suspected to be caused by the conversion of glucose sugars into sorbitol inside our eye cells. Sorbitol cannot pass through the cell walls, so once inside, it stays trapped. It then attracts extra sodium and water, that interfere with the osmotic balance that controls the passage of nutrients and oxygen into these cells. Potassium, magnesium, glutathione and amino acids are lost, causing the cells to die.

Other causes of cataracts could be damage from the ultra-violet rays of the sun, excess of antihistamines, corticosteroids, cigarette smoke and eye infections. The drug tetracycline has been know to make the eye-lens more susceptible to damage from ultra violet rays; therefore, take precautions to avoid sunlight when using this prescription. Low calcium levels and heavy metal poisoning also have been know to contribute to cataracts. You should try to detox your body from heavy metal poisoning.

Increasing your trace mineral intake can help to chelate these from the body.

To prevent or reduce the formation of cataracts, it is essential to increase levels of glycine, cysteine and glutamine amino acids in the eye lens. Also beneficial to prevent cataracts is the intake of essential crystalloid electrolyte trace minerals, vitamins A,B,C and E as well as two specific bioflavonoids, Quercetin and Naringen, found in grapefruit, broccoli, blue-green algae, and summer squash. Increase your intake of vitamin C. The University of Western Ontario studies showed that 1000-2500 mg. of vitamin C reduced the incidence of cataracts by 70%. Herbal treatments for cataracts include bilberry, eyebright, goldenseal root powder and rue. Homeopathic remedies are Euphrasia, Carbo-Animales, Phosphorus, Apis and Silicea.

Macular degeneration and light sensitivity. Macular degeneration is a retinal disorder that obscures central vision among an estimated four million Americans. Most people have heard that taking quantities of vitamin A (beta-carotene) can protect your eyes. Beta-carotene is only one class of carotenoids that are involved in the maintenance of the visual system. The other is xanthophylls (leutin and zeaxanthin), which are found in spinach, kale, collards, spirulina, amaranth, marigold flower petals and mustard greens. They are necessary as light filters for the eye. People with macular degeneration have been found to be lacking in proper levels of lutein and zeaxanthin.

As with most things nature has designed, there should be balance. If you are taking quantities of beta-carotene rich foods and supplements, then you should balance with leutin and/or zeaxanthin. These ingredients are extracted from marigold flower petals for use in supplements. Because of the vulnerability of the central retina to sun damage when lutein is in short supply, it is strongly advised that all multi-vitamins that provide beta-carotene include an equal amount of lutein. This is particularly important for individuals at risk for macular degeneration (smokers, postmenopausal females and those with light eye color), who should actually consume more lutein. Some people who supplement with lutein and zeaxanthin report reduced glare and visual fatigue, better night vision, and less dependency upon sunglasses. It does take about two months after beginning supplementation to notice a difference, so be patient.

Glaucoma. This disease is caused where internal pressure increases, causing vision difficulties, and even blindness. The pressure causes the optic nerve to atrophy and globe of the eye to enlarge. Initial signs of glaucoma is experiencing halos around lights, mild headaches, impaired ability to adjust to dark and a frequent need to alter eyeglass prescriptions. There are few agreements into the causes of glaucoma, although many studies link this disease to Glutathione deficiencies. This has also been implicated in age-related Macular degeneration, which is the result of free radical damage to the nerve fibers that transmit signals to the brain.

Holistic practitioners recommend an increased intake of amino acids, including Glutathione. This should be taken side by side with a good mineral supplement that not only can improve the body's balance, but can help against free radical damage. Vitamins C, E and the bioflavonoid rutin are also beneficial. The New York State Journal of Medicine reported a study of 26 patients with pressure on the eye. Seventeen out of twenty six patients reported a pressure drop of 15% when give prescribed dosages of rutin.

Oxygen therapy is important for cellular support; therefore, taking a supplement containing oxygen would be helpful. Herbal treatments include Ginkgo biloba and huckleberry. Bilberry should not be used for this condition, as it is thought to further increase pressure on the eye.

GOUT.

This is a disease that causes sudden and severe attacks of pain, tenderness, redness and swelling in some joints. Uric acid crystals build up in the joint, causing the pain and swelling. Uric acid is a substance that normally forms when the body breaks down certain proteins and circulates their associated waste products throughout the body. As a normal course of metabolism, it usually is dissolved in the blood, and passes through the kidneys and out into the urine. However, in people with gout, this process does not occur completely, and excess crystals build up in the joints.

Mineral deficiencies can prevent the body from flushing out excess uric acid, reducing the kidney's inability to process the acid before it settles out of solution. An attack of gout can be triggered by drinking excess alcohol, eating foods high in purines, surgery, joint injuries and over use of drugs such as thiazide diuretic which causes a potassium deficiency. Avoiding wine, anchovies, beer, beef, gravy and liver are dietary prescriptions delivered by most doctors, along with prescription drugs to reduce the pain and swelling. Natural methods include drinking black cherry juice, and applying a poultice of chopped fresh onions on the affected area daily. Homeopathic remedies can assist in the removal of uric acid from the affected areas of the body. Rhus toxicodendron 10x taken once daily or as needed, normalizes the elimination of the uric acid and may relieve the pain.

Rhododendron caucasicum extract has been successfully used to treat gout for many centuries in the former USSR. According to the results of clinical trials, in 320 volunteers, the extract of Rhododendron increased the discharge of Uric acid by more than 35-60% relieving pain after only a few hours *(Samartzev, Aushev and Israelov, 1065, Russian Clinical Research, Academy of Sciences)*. They found that if they continued the treatment over several days, the symptoms of the illness significantly decreased.

Other treatments for gout include yucca and devil's claw leaves, chaparral, fresh pipsissewa herb, fresh juniper berry, fresh stinging nettle leaf, burdock and ginkgo. You can also chew grains of mustard seeds and drink a strong infusion of elder buds in the morning and evening.

HEART DISEASE.

This illness attacks more people during the mid-life and later years, and it would be nice if we could give our bodies a better defense. Watching your diet and exercising have always been the rule, but many times that is not enough. Many heart attacks come from clogged arteries, meaning the blood sticks to the arterial walls, eventually forming a blockage called arteriosclerosis. Normally smooth, the walls may become damaged because of environmental toxins or free radical damage, resulting in the blood sticking to those injured areas. These stuck cells then may release growth hormones, and slowly get larger, picking up LDL (low density lipoprotein) cholesterol and becoming "fat". Eventually they will block blood flow to the heart. Bioflavonoids are a beneficial supplement to guard against plaque build up.

Aged garlic extract can also offer some protection to this process. Dr. Manfred Steins, Brown University and Dr. Robert I-San Lin, Ph.D., discovered that aged garlic extract and its active compounds are potent inhibitors of platelet adhesion. The only other substance to have this property is tocopherol, a form of Vitamin E. While aspirin may inhibit platelet aggregation, it cannot prevent platelet adhesion. Aged garlic extract has shown it does both and without side effects. Other studies have concluded that the active compounds of aged garlic extract (S-allyl cysteine and S-ally mercaptocysteine) inhibit the growth of cells which could eventually block the artery. Aged garlic extract also has been found to lower LDL cholesterol, and suggested that it may also slow the body's cholesterol synthesis. Even though Kyolic® has had the majority of studies conducted on garlic's healthy benefits, Lictwer Pharmacy of Germany (makers of KWAI garlic) has also had numerous studies performed on its cholesterol-lowering effects.

Also beneficial for protecting the heart from damage are the herbs hawthorn berry and cayenne. Supplementing your diet with essential fatty acids in the form of flax seed can reduce the build up of arterial plaque. Electrolyte balance must be present to have any treatment be effective. Supplementing your diet with crystalloid electrolytes can make the difference in the speed of any recovery.

Artherosclerosis (occlusion of passageways through the arteries) actually begins when the smooth muscle cells within the middle layer of the artery wall lose self control and begin reproducing themselves at an accelerated rate. A lump forms within the artery wall that eventually breaks through the inner lining of the artery. This broken spot reveals a lump of tangled muscle cells and collagen, for in the process of over-replication, the muscle cells have also generated more binding collagen than needed. It is this unbridled growth of muscle cells that leads many researchers to refer to atherosclerosis as arterial cancer.

These renegade muscle cells are brought to this elevated level because of sticky blood platelets. These are caused by an over abundance of omega-6 EFAs not balanced by omega-3's, and/or the benzopyrene and tars from cigarette smoke and/or LDL cholesterol which causes the muscle cells to choke on their own growth factor, thus activating over-growth. A specific antioxidant, tocotrienol which is a close cousin to vitamin E, can reduce the synthesis of LDL cholesterol by the liver. Along with vitamin E, it activates the release of transforming growth factor beta from muscle cells within the artery walls, therefore working directly against the action of the LDL cholesterol. The tocotrienols are more effective at lowering LDL levels than vitamin E alone. Tocotrienols are found along with vitamin E, in grains such as barley, soybeans, rice, amaranth and others.

HOT FLASHES.

Night (or day) sweats are not really fever-like temperature rises, although try telling that to most women who are in the midst of taking off their sweaters...again! They occur when there are changes in the diameter of the blood vessels near the skin surface, making only the skin temperature rise. When levels of adrenaline and cortisone are increased in the body, such as during darkness, hot flashes result. Low sodium can also cause an increase in adrenaline. Therefore, taking a crystalloid trace mineral solution will help. Hot flashes can be triggered by dietary habits, alcohol, tobacco, coffee, spicy foods and eating large meals.

Pantothenic Acid is useful to help stress and is necessary for adrenal function; therefore, if hot flashes persist, try adding this supplement to your diet. Good news for women who carry a little extra fat comes from the menopausal practitioners. Because an adrenal hormone can be converted to estrogen and stored in body fat, it seems that thin women seem to suffer more during menopause than those who are heavier. Don't take this as an excuse to gorge yourself, because obese women are high risk for uterine and breast cancer due to too much estrogen production. Natural progesterone supplementation, from the organic wild yam, can balance this condition.

The production of progesterone from cholesterol is dependent on adequate thyroid function, plus vitamin A (fish oil source is best) and certain enzymes. Adding natural progesterone, along with vitamin A and enzymes may help to control night sweats. Using estrogen alone to diminish hot flashes is like using a drug. It keeps the body in a continuous state of excitation causing increased levels of adrenaline. It works because a hot flash occurs when adrenal levels are in a relaxed state, after an increase. Like keeping yourself awake with coffee, estrogen keeps you in an "up" state so the adrenaline levels never go down. This may prevent hot flashes, but can also create numerous side effects.

Vitamin E (combined with vitamin C as a carrier) can reduce hot flashes and also improve circulation, as well as help prevent varicose veins and blood clots. Recommended dosages should come from a physician or a naturopathic doctor, as overdoses may cause some side effects especially in diabetics or people taking blood thinners or high blood pressure medicine.

Evening primrose oil, a source of the essential fatty acid GLA (gamma-linolenic acid), is necessary for hormone production and has been successful at reducing the effects of hot flashes. Omega 3 and Omega 6 fatty acids, found in certain oils or ground flax seed, are beneficial in reducing hot flashes. Homeopathic remedies include Lachesis for severe hot flashes and Pulsatilla for milder ones.

Herbal remedies include combinations of dong quai, ginseng, hawthorn berries, black cohosh, wild yam root, chaste tree berry and licorice root, compounded sage, motherwort and peppermint and compounded vitex/alfalfa. These herbs are good for all around menopausal symptom relief. Some have found that drinking a tea containing sage, lady's mantle and horsetail relieves symptoms. Others advise taking a combination of cod liver oil, vitamin E with C, evening primrose oil supplements and gamma oryzanol (within rice bran oil). Examine if foods trigger hot flashes, and avoid eating those that cause symptoms. Many find that eating sugary foods or fruit can trigger a hot flash several minutes later.

INSOMNIA.

Sleeplessness is a common malady for people whose immune systems have been compromised either through stress, illness, depression, anxiety, hypoglycemia, over-use of certain drugs or poor diet. Sleeping pills are only "Band-Aids". They do not cure the underlying cause of the insomnia. Chronic loss of sleep leads to fatigue, anxiety, poor performance and depression. Several processes affect sleep. Disruption of melatonin levels produced by the pineal gland can cause irregular sleep patterns. Melatonin supplements may help some people sleep, but others may find it keeps them awake. Herbal sleep remedies are far safer than drug type sleeping pills and come with no side effects.

Meditation to reduce stress can help if done on a regular basis. Following the recommendations for minerals, enzymes and essential fatty acid supplementation is essential to supporting the immune system and reducing stress. As mentioned several times in this book, amino acid support is key in providing the brain's neurotransmitters to function properly. When supported, they will better be able to turn off your thought process and let you go to sleep. Lecithin, which helps memory, can also be beneficial in treating insomnia. The herbs ginseng, ginkgo and hawthorn can be soothing and calming.

Depending on the cause of the insomnia, you can try soothing music, and soaking your feet in a solution of hot water and vinegar. Avoid eating big meals and stimulant types of foods before retiring. You can also make a brew of one teaspoon of plain gelatin in one cup of boiling water, and take two teaspoons of this with dinner. Warm milk may be beneficial, as it releases natural tryptophan. Herbs that may help are Valerian, a safe sedative, passion flower which has a tranquilizing effect, chamomile that improves relaxation, and kava kava which is an anti-spasmodic and soothes nerves. Skullcap, hops and celery seed are also used in herbal sleep formulas as well as compounded elixir of passionflower, compounded skullcap/St. John's wort, hope, vervain, valerian, catnip, peppermint and golden seal. Oatseed is soothing and supporting of the nervous system, and alleviates depression, insomnia and anxiety. Royal jelly is effective for insomnia. Biochemic remedies include Nat. Phos. (Sodium Phosphate) in alternation with Nat. Sulph. (Sodium Sulphate) when due to digestive disturbances, and Kali. Phos. (Potassium Phosphate), when insomnia stems from nervousness or over-excitement.

MEMORY.

The brain's remarkable ability to perceive and perform, remember and learn, is severely challenged by today's social and physical environment. These factors accelerate the decline in nerve cell activity that normally occurs with age. Phosphatidyl Serine (PS) is a phospholipid which forms an essential part in every human cell, but it is particularly concentrated in the membranes of nerve cells. Unlike other cells in the body, nerve cells do not reproduce. Instead, they repair and rebuild themselves, using proteins called Nerve Growth Factor (NGF). PS enhances the synthesis and reception of NGF and supports brain functions that tend to diminish with age. PS also may be related to the body's response to stress, as taking a PS supplement appears to produce fewer stress hormones in response to exercise-induced stress. PS may have the potential to minimize a common problem in today's world-stress induced memory lapse.

Amino acids are necessary to keep the brain's neurotransmitters firing properly. Part of the aging brain's failing memory problem is recalling information. Supporting the brain with DL-phenylalanine and L-Glutamine, two key amino acids, will provide the ammunition the body needs to repair or rebuild failing neural signals. Stress can deplete these amino acids, as well as insufficient diet, alcohol and drug abuse. In addition to failing memory, lack of neurotransmitter support can cause depression, fatigue, anxiety and feelings of hopelessness normally associated with 'just getting old'. These key amino acids are found in cold-water white fish, or available through supplements.

Lecithin is produced by our livers, and is a major part of the brain. It is made up of Choline, Linoleic acid and Inositol, which are successful in crossing the blood-brain barrier necessary to nourish brain cells. In his book, *Boost Your Brainpower*, Dr. Julian Whitaker, M.D. explains that lecithin is the major source of the neurotransmitter acetylcholine which determines human behavior, and is the most important substance in nerve transmission. It is particularly needed by the brain for repair and maintenance. As we age, acetylcholine levels decline, leading to a reduction in both short and long-term memory. As an essential fatty acid it also helps lower blood pressure and regulate cholesterol levels. Deficiencies can hamper the proper operation of the brain. In *Prescriptions for Nutritional Healing,* James Balch, M.D. tells us that the protective sheaths surrounding the brain are composed of lecithin, as are the muscles and nerves. Therefore, maintaining adequate levels of lecithin can help to reduce the mental symptoms associated with aging. Extracted from egg yolks and soybeans, lecithin is easy to come by as a supplement.

Herbal suggestions start with ginkgo biloba, which helps relax the muscles in our blood vessels, allowing more blood and oxygen to get to the brain. This is a primary brain and mental energy stimulant, that increases both peripheral and cerebral circulation through vasodilation. It also is effective for vertigo, dizziness and ringing in the ears. Newer research suggests that ginkgo counteracts the sexual side effects of antidepressants such as Prozac and Zoloft. In addition to ginkgo, herbs such as anise, periwinkle, St. John's wort, gotu kola, Siberian ginseng, wild oats, Chinese fo-ti and rosemary leaves are helpful for memory retention.

Dietary regimes should avoid allergenic foods such as sugar, wheat and dairy. Aspartame sweetener should be avoided at all costs. It changes dopamine levels in the brain affecting memory, speech, vision and inducing headaches. Flax should be consumed daily, as it is high in essential fatty acids that are a key component to the brain. If the cause of the memory loss is attributed to heavy metal accumulation, you can chelate the toxins out with a good crystalloid electrolyte mineral complex. Proper diagnosis of heavy metal storage can be determined through a hair analysis.

Many emotional problems associated with memory failure can be treated with flower remedies. The use of flower remedies can be effective in cases where the feelings of discouragement, failure, insecurity, lethargy and frustration are present. People with a lack of concentration may be helped by clematis. Those who are discouraged can be helped by gentian. Motivation may be bolstered through wild rose. These remedies are commonly administered through tinctures placed under the tongue, and work within minutes.

OSTEOPOROSIS.

This condition happens when the body fails to utilize calcium, which leeches out of the bone. It is marked by the appearance of small holes in the bones, and a generalized thinning of bony tissue. Osteoporosis affects over 28 million Americans, and is one of the top three most life-threatening diseases in the U.S., affecting both women and men. After age 35, when peak bone mass is reached, the male's decreasing rate of bone density averages about 1% per year, with women experiencing considerably higher rates.

Osteoporosis is not an estrogen-deficiency disease. Bone-forming cells come in two kinds: Osteoclasts dissolve old bone, leaving empty spaces readying it for new bone growth; osteoblasts move into these spaces to build the new bone. Too much estrogen stimulates the osteoclasts, resulting in bone loss. In this condition, the osteoblasts which have progesterone receptors, are prevented from building back the bone. In balancing the estrogen by adding progesterone, you will actually create the environment for the osteoblasts to do their job; this can prevent or reverse the bone loss and the osteoporosis condition.

Osteoporosis is indicated by pain, especially in the lower back, frequent broken bones, loss of height, and is sometimes linked to other disorders associated with hyper-parathyroidism. If we begin at an early age, we can prevent osteoporosis. The normal time for rebuilding of solid bone is ten to twelve years. Rebuilding of the spongy bone is two to three years, with five to ten percent of our bone being replaced by this process each year. As we age, more bone is broken down than is created. This could be a function of the xeno-estrogens from our environment, causing an over-estrogen condition. Drug therapies currently given to prevent blood vessels from breaking down the bone, may actually produce an overabundance of new bone that competes for space with the old bone. This bone disparity creates more risk of fracture.

There are better ways to prevent bone loss. If we have built a good quantity of bone mass during our younger years, our bone loss will be less. Therefore, it is important to start being concerned about osteoporosis well before you reach fifty. Using a royal jelly supplement can help by accelerating the formation of bone tissue, and by keeping a balanced pH, as discussed in an earlier chapter, you can create an essential condition for bone-making. Most people think that by just adding calcium, you will build up your defense against osteoporosis. This is not the case. Magnesium must be taken as well, because it is a carrier for the calcium on its trip to the bone. If too much calcium is taken, it will actually cause a magnesium deficiency in the body, resulting in nervousness, fatigue, heart palpitations and depression. Excess calcium also can work to prevent this calcium from getting into the bones at all.

Do not eat quantities of dairy (better to substitute with rice or almond milk products), without supplementing your diet with magnesium rich foods such as kale, seeds, nuts, barley and wheatgrass and dark green vegetables. Avoid sugar, sodas containing phosphoric acid, and the diuretic Lasix, as they all contribute to leeching calcium from the body. During and after menopause the body's ability to hold on to calcium declines, and bone-calcium loss can be intense for as long as ten years after menopause.

Osteoporosis is a repercussion of imbalance. The equilibrium of specific minerals in the blood, including calcium, is critical, and the body has special mechanisms to ensure their constancy. Calcium's availability fluctuates all the time. The bones act as a bank which the body can draw on if dietary calcium is low, or return to when the absorption is high. This system can be disrupted by dieting and inadequate nutrition, excesses of certain non-foods and processed foods, unremitting stress, and long-term use of certain drugs. It is generally not until menopause that the process of bone loss becomes accelerated to a critical point, due to the fluctuations in estrogen/progesterone.

Trace minerals or electrolytes are involved in the health of the glands and the production of the hormones that control calcium's use in the body. All the body's functions are sensitive to changes in mineral balance. For example, if the body is out of homeostasis, calcium deficiency will occur, no matter how high the calcium intake. A high intake of calcium may disrupt the body's levels of zinc, iron and manganese. These minerals also influence calcium's absorption. In order to absorb and use calcium, the body needs vitamin D, magnesium and trace minerals, including copper. Too much vitamin A, E or potassium will upset calcium metabolism, and decrease its availability.

When our bodies are low in calcium, they can borrow from reserves in the bones. Magnesium is also stored in the bones, which won't give up as much of it as calcium. Instead, our bodies take magnesium from muscles. Without enough magnesium in muscles to counterbalance the stimulating effect of calcium, they stiffen up or contract at will, resulting in cramps, irritability, twitching or tremors.

Boron is a naturally occurring trace mineral that should be part of any calcium/magnesium supplement. It decreases the urinary excretion of calcium and magnesium, and increases blood levels of estrogen, vitamin D and other hormones. Boron, found mainly in fruit, raises serum estrogen levels in post menopausal women, thereby reducing calcium and magnesium loss. Silica influences the uptake of calcium in the bones. Silica also has the wonderful advantage (to women especially) of strengthening nails and causing them to grow. Vitamin D has shown to reduce the incidence of hip fractures in post-menopausal women. In a study at Tufts University, women who took 400 I.U. of vitamin D daily has less bone loss during the winter months (lack of adequate sunlight), than women who took a placebo.

Exercise influences bone density, and trace minerals aid the absorption of nutrients (100 percent). Together, along with estrogen/progesterone balance, they make a winning team of preventing osteoporosis. In our chapter on fitness we give several bone building exercises. Stay away from sugar, as it inhibits calcium absorption, alters insulin metabolism, which affects calcium metabolism, and facilitates loss of vitamin B6 levels, which upset magnesium. It also robs the body of trace minerals so rapidly and thoroughly, that it upsets every physical process and increases the long-term risk of osteoporosis.

It is also essential that you supplement your diet with enzymes to guard against osteoporosis. The protease enzyme is important in calcium metabolism, and plant enzymes aid proper digestion, necessary for the nutrient extraction needed for healthy bones. When shopping for enzymes, make sure they say 'plant source' on the bottle or you will not be getting the full complement of enzymes.

Isoflavone used in Japan and Europe, is a non-hormonal agent from plant bioflavonoids and other constituents. This supplement increases bone mineral density significantly, as shown in clinical trials. In as short a time as three to nine months, bone density increased by 2 to 9% when using 600 mg/day of Isoflavone. It also has shown to inhibit the formation of osteoclasts, reduce bone resorption and stimulate the formation of bone-building osteoblasts. In a long term clinical trial using Isoflavone as a supplement on 75 diagnosed patients suffering from osteoporosis, 58% experienced pain relief in four weeks, 57% felt better in three weeks, and 87% had good results in 48 weeks.

Herbal treatments include drinking a tea three times a day containing the following ingredients: wild oats, nettles, marshmallow root, yellow dock and horsetail (silica). Osteoporosis must be prevented through proper diet and supplementation, as we have described in another chapter of this book. The wise addition of bee pollen, royal jelly, calcium and magnesium,

Vitamin C, D, K and trace elements, especially Boron, will help to guard against this disease.

PANIC ATTACKS.

Fear and anxiety can become a real handicap for women in menopause, who now become afraid of elevators, airplanes, stuffy rooms and the like. Flower remedies in a combination of aspen, mimulus, blackberry, cherry plum, red chestnut and rock rose, along with garlic, give almost immediate relief from panic attacks. Herbal treatments include compounded elixir of passionflower, compounded skullcap/St. John's wort, compounded melissa. Probotanixx's *An Shen (includes Zizyphus, Polygonum, Albizzia, Hoelen, Cnidium, Schizandra, Coptis, Anemarrhena, Rehmannia, Licorice). Homeopathic remedies include Gelsemium sempervirens. Bee pollen has had a relaxing effect on some people, and may help with anxiety. Also refraining from intake of sugars, caffeine, alcohol or other stimulants will reduce the triggers that cause these attacks.

PARKINSON'S DISEASE.

This is a serious, degenerative central nervous system condition, characterized by a slowly spreading tremor, muscular weakness, speech interference, and body rigidity. It occurs in about one in two hundred people over the age of 50. Contributing factors to the onset of Parkinson's are hyperthyroidism, aluminum/heavy metal toxicity, pesticide residues, and anger, which thwarts the body's ability to let go of toxins. Poor diet influences symptoms, especially when foods ingested are high in chemical additives and excitotoxins. Also implicated are red wine, foods containing nitrate and nitrite preservatives, caffeine and drugs that cause blood vessels to dilate.

Similar to people diagnosed with attention deficit disorder symptoms, scientific results indicate that there is a connection between low levels of the hormone dopamine, and those suffering from Parkinson's disease .The basal ganglia help control body

126

movement and they rely on dopamine, which is transported from the substantia nigra. In Parkinson's disease, degeneration of the substantia nigra means that the basal ganglia receive reduced amounts of dopamine. Professor Zakir Ramazanov, Ph.D., explains further. "In the normal brain, the levels of dopamine and acetylcholine are evenly balanced. In Parkinson's disease, the levels of dopamine are reduced and acetylcholine is abundant. Several studies have shown that extract of Rhodeola Rosea (Siberian plant extract) naturally stimulate the level of dopamine in the brain. Rhodeola Rosea is in a class of herbs called adaptogens, which help the body adapt to demands that are placed on it reducing stress. Studies have shown it improves brain-cell activity, and helps the body to use oxygen more efficiently. This oxygenation process increases blood levels of specific brain chemicals that relax us, and reduces the nerve-jangling effects caused by stress hormones. Administration of Rhodeola Rosea to Parkinsonian patients was shown to be very beneficial."

A combination of herbs traditionally used for cancer therapy has recently been adapted as a supportive treatment for Parkinson disease. This formula, known as Essiac, consists of sheep sorrel, burdock root, turkey rhubarb and slippery elm bark.

Excitotoxins, a group of natural excitatory amino acids that may cause sensitive neurons to die, are also thought to contribute to the onset of Parkinson disease. Glutamate and aspartate are neurotransmitters normally found in the brain and spinal chord. They are two of the most common transmitters of chemicals in the brain, but when their levels become excessive not only do they become deadly to the neurons containing glutamine receptors but they kill the nerve cells connected to these neurons. This can create a domino effect, wherein brain cells in another location my begin to die, producing a fine tremor of the hands and rigid, plastic-like movements of the body parts. Parkinson's disease does not manifest until over 80-90% of the neurons in the involved nuclei have died. This takes years of assault from the excitotoxin ingestion to accomplish.

Excitotoxins created artificially appear in monosodium glutamate (MSG), hydrolyzed vegetable protein, cysteine supplements and aspartame (Nutrasweet). Hydrolyzed vegetable protein (HVP) is used as a major ingredient for soups and many other savory foods. It is made by boiling vegetables for several hours in a vat of sulfuric acid which is then neutralized with caustic soda. The sludge is scraped off the top and dried to form a brown powder to which "free" MSG is then often added. The end product is a substance high in three excitotoxins, glutamate, aspartate and cystoic acid. MSG in the "free" or separated form within the flavor enhancer that causes many people to develop migraine headaches, joint pain and other negative reactions.

Aspartame is composed of neuroexcitatory amino acids and methyl alcohol, and acts as a mind-altering drug in disturbing the chemical balance of the brain. It obstructs the production of serotonin, a key neurotransmitter and affects brain phenylalanine and tyrosine levels. According to Mary Nash Stoddard, Aspartame Consumer Safety Network, Inc., "that although the amino acids in aspartame are natural, when produced synthetically in a laboratory, do not behave in the same manner as when found in nature. Aspartame is a prescription for disaster." Reactions have been documented such as headaches, seizures, mental aberrations, urinary disturbances, and chronic neurological disorders. Symptoms of overuse of Aspartame have even been misdiagnosed as Multiple Sclerosis. To prevent against Parkinson's disease and reduce its acceleration, people should absolutely avoid these ingredients. For more information on excitotoxins, read *Excitotoxins, The Taste That Kills,* by Russell Blaylock, M.D.

A word of caution for those people who ingest excitotoxins. Evidence has shown that *prescription* L-dopa therapy should not be administered at the same time. The prescription L-dopa can actually speed up the progress of the disease when combined with excitotoxins. Also, when L-dopa is given, it is necessary to avoid multi-vitamins that contain vitamin B6 as that particular vitamin blocks L-dopa to the brain. L-dopa is not to be confused with natural treatments that create the body's production of dopamine. L-dopa is one of a series of precursors, or building blocks, used by the body to manufacture the neurotransmitters dopamine, norepinephrine and epinephrine. L-dopa stimulates both the dopamine and the norepinephrine systems of the brain. L-dopa is found naturally in the human body, but it occurs in some foods including Velvet beans (Mucuna Pruriens) a very potent and rare Ayurvedic herb. L-dopa is one of the few substances the crosses the blood barrier and converts into dopamine. It supplements the body with any of the precursors in the sequence of phenylalanine, tyrosine and dopa, resulting in greater brain levels of norepinephrine, a major neurotransmitter that creates feelings of happiness and reduces depression.

It is important to support the nerves and their neurotransmitters. This is best done with an essential fatty acid supplement, or by adding flax to your diet. You also need to provide your body with the key amino acids that form neurotransmitters. DL-phenylalanine and L-Glutamine can be found in cold-water white fish and certain amino acid supplements. Many times tremors are aggravated because the brain isn't transmitting the proper signal, due to 'faulty' or depleted neurotransmitters. In Parkinson's victims, stress and bottled-up emotions play havoc with our neurotransmitters, creating a dire need for amino acid support.

For those people suffering from early stages of Parkinson's disease, it would be wise to take a look at your lifestyle. Eliminating chemicals from your environment along with excitotoxins in your foods, should be the first step to fighting the disease. Natural cleaners and furnishings, along with organic foods, should be your only consideration. A hair-mineral analysis can confirm any heavy metal concentrations in your body. Taking a good cyrstalloid electrolyte supplement will assist in the chelation (removal) of these toxins from your body. Avoid anything with aluminum in it such as deodorant, baking powder, cooking utensils and many calcium supplements (ask the manufacturer).

PROSTATE PROBLEMS.

The prostate is a large male gland that lies just below the neck of the bladder and around the top of the urinary tract. The primary function of the prostate is to help the semen move through the urethra during ejaculation. Because of this, it enlarges during sexual arousal. If there is prolonged arousal without ejaculation, prostate pressure on the testicles becomes very uncomfortable (commonly referred to as blue balls.) Symptoms associated with enlarged prostate include frequent, painful desire to urinate, reduced flow of urine, incontinence and in extreme cases, fever, lower back pain, insomnia and fatigue. Accompanying symptoms associated with sexual dysfunction are impotence, loss of libido and possible painful ejaculation.

Obesity and hormonal changes are two well known causes of prostate enlargement. Disorders usually begin after age 35. By age 50, over 25% of all men have enlarged prostate and by age 80 the numbers grow to 80%. A diet high in saturated fats and low in the beneficial essential fatty acids puts people at the greatest risk. Factored in as causes are hormonal imbalances, low fiber diets, spicy foods, and excessive use of alcohol and caffeine, eating meat from animals injected with hormones, prostaglandin depletion, an exhausted lymph system from chronic usage of antihistamines, a lack of exercise, zinc deficiency and venereal disease. Enlargement of the prostate may be caused by an enzyme, testosterone reductase, which interacts with testosterone and produces di-hydrotestosterone (DHT). Alcohol, especially beer, elevates levels of DHT in the body, and thus can be a contributing factor. The herb saw palmetto supports prostate health by promoting a reduction in DHT in tissue by over 40%. It balances the body's hormones to block painful prostate enlargement, and can be an effective natural treatment. Pygeum africanum, an herb, also lowers DHT levels by blocking cholesterol production.

Vasectomies also lay suspect in contributing to prostate problems. Science has long debated whether risk of prostate cancer is a result of vasectomy (the contraceptive procedure that severs or seals off the vessel that carries sperm from the testes.) New studies on two large group of men show that vasectomies increase risk of prostate cancer. In one study of 73,000 men between 1986 and 1990, those with vasectomies had a 66% greater risk of prostate cancer. In a separate study, vasectomies increased the risk of prostate cancer by 56%. After a vasectomy, sperm build up in the sealed off vas deferens. The body reabsorbs these cells which confuses the immune system, making it less alert to tumor cells. It also causes the body's defenses to mount a response against its own tissue. In addition, a vasectomy affects hormone secretions in the testes, and lowers prostatic fluid. When the natural movement of sperm and hormones are artificially prevented, numerous health problems may arise.

Men who have chronic constipation may create prostate problems. In a healthy person there is space between the colon and the prostate. Constipation causes the colon to swell and push against the prostate. If this condition is chronic, bacteria from the colon can migrate through the muscles and mucous membranes of the colon and penetrate the stroma tissue surrounding the prostate. This condition is called prostatitis. Kenneth Yasny Ph.D., in his book *Put Hemorrhoids and Constipation Behind You* gives suggestions that may alleviate constipation. Eat moist foods and drink lots of water to help waste move through our system. Eat high fiber foods that absorb moisture, and grease your intestines with polyunsaturated or monounsaturated oils.

Unfortunately, a cardinal rule in natural prostate recovery is abstinence. Sexual intercourse irritates the prostate and delays the repair process. Treating prostate problems with drug therapy comes with a list of side effects that can include loss of libido and decreased potency. To naturally reduce inflammation of the prostate, you should avoid alcohol, caffeine, carbonated drinks, tomato juice, fried and refined foods and red meat. A deficiency in zinc may lead to changes in the size, structure and function of the prostate. Because of its very high zinc content, Bee pollen can have great value in healing the prostate gland when used as supplement.

A specialty diet is included in Linda Rector Page's *Healthy Healing* book that includes high fiber, whole grains, low fats and a cleansing with lemon juice and water. She mentions many herbal treatments. These include saw palmetto (prevents the breakdown of testosterone to DHT), echinacea/goldenseal (for inflammation), white oak (to shrink swollen prostate), hydrangea (reduce sediment), garlic (an anti-ineffective), and damiana (wards off infection). Nettles are also frequently used as they inhibit the binding of DHT to attachment sites on the prostate membrane, therefore diminishing its effect on prostrate enlargement.

Saw palmetto is a natural steroid source herb with tissue-building and gland-stimulating properties to tonify and strengthen the male reproductive system. It is a primary herb for male impotence, low libido, and prostate health. The potency is increased when combined with another herb called damiana, which also helps to increase sperm count. Sabal Serrulata, the homeopathic form of saw palmetto, is formulated to address the irritability of the genito-urinary organs. It promotes nutrition and tissue building, and is very valuable in treating prostatic enlargement. Pygeum africanum is especially effective in inhibiting the production of prostaglandins in the prostate. It helps with inflammation, blood cholesterol and excess fluid in the prostate. For men with an ailing prostate gland, the herb ginseng appears to help healing and normalization of function.

SEXUAL DYSFUNCTION.

Emotional symptoms leading to sexual inadequacies may not be caused by mental anguish, but can be the result of dietary deficiencies and environmental assaults on the body. Those people who experience a low sex drive typically have symptoms of Vitamin B6 (pyridoxine) deficiency, according to studies by Dr. Pat Bermond at the medical clinic of the University of Reims in France. Symptoms of this deficiency show up as cracks around the nose or mouth, a common side effect of drinking alcohol. Before you seek psychological help, you may want to analyze your lifestyle and eating habits.

Drug use, refined foods, sugar, caffeine, alcohol and tobacco all may diminish sexual desire and contribute to depression and stress. Any substance that creates a high must eventually result in a low. It's this low that affects the body and lessens the sex drive. Sexual desire originates in the brain, and it must be nourished.

A lack of healthy fats (essential fatty acids), as well as a protein-deficient diet, may inhibit brain activity, thus contributing to loss of sexual interest. Dietary changes may be all that is needed to restore libido. The saw palmetto herb can act as a mild aphrodisiac for men. The herb, damiana, when used in combination with other herbs, has also been used as an aphrodisiac and to improve the sexual ability of the enfeebled and aged male. It is thought to work by slightly irritating the urethra, thereby producing increased sensitivity of the penis, and increasing sexual desire.

Velvet antlers, when harvested (by a method that doesn't hurt the elk/deer) at a certain time of the year, becomes a very potent source of hormones, minerals, amino acids and enzymes as well as cartilage. Elk and deer in their natural setting eat a variety of herbs, including ginseng, which is considered an aphrodisiac. Velvet antlers contain both the male and female hormone precursors. One of the hormones, testosterone, is extremely important in that it stimulates growth and sexual potency in both men and women. Higher testosterone, levels found in women elicit a greater interest in sex, and increased orgasms.

In aging men, as testosterone levels decline, there is a resulting commensurate loss of sex drive, premature ejaculation and the inability to maintain an erection. The hormone called leuteinizing hormone (LH) that is secreted by the pituitary gland, gives the signal for testosterone to be produced. Velvet antlers have high levels of LH and testosterone which stimulate the male testicle to convert cholesterol to testosterone.

Chinese doctors have used antler velvet for male incontinence, prostatic problems, and enlarged prostates for thousands of years. This may be attributed to other parts of the antler, such as the anti-inflammatory prostaglandins and the anti-inflammatory portions of the cartilage. For women, besides helping with frigidity and infertility, the antlers contain a high amount of calcium, useful in preventing osteoporosis. It may also help in the treatment of menstrual disorders.

Three herbs from the Amazon can act as aphrodisiacs, and have been used for impotence: marapuama, catuaba and cajueiro with marapuama being most effective for erectile dysfunctions. Chewing on ginseng root daily helps, along with taking the herbs damiana, *Fo-Ti, gotu-kola, sarsaparilla, saw palmetto, and *Shou Wu Chih formula (Radix Polygoni Multifori). Ginseng enhances male vitality, especially when in combination with herbs like sarsaparilla and damiana. This herb also enhances nitric oxide synthesis, regulating the muscular tone of blood vessels to control blood flow to the penis, similar to the effect of popular drugs such as Viagra.

Bee pollen can improve sperm production and increase sexual libido. Prostate inflammation can be helped by compounded saw palmetto, fresh thuja leaf, compounded echinacea, Pau d'arco, jatoba, burdock, cornsilk, couch grass, uva ursi, buchu leaves, juniper berries and marshmallow. Homeopathic treatments include Mag. Phos. (Magnesium Phosphate) and Nat. Sulph. (Sodium Phosphate).

Flower remedies are extremely useful for treating the emotion surrounding sexual dysfunction. In cases of sexual inadequacies, feelings of failure, insecurity, irritation, and frustration may be lessened with the help of flower remedies. People with feelings of inadequacy may be helped by flower essences of elm, larch, larkspur, saguaro cactus and wild mountain iris. Feelings of frustration can be helped by chaparral, daffodil, impatiens, lotus, morning glory, potentilla, wild mountain iris and willow. These preparations are commonly administered by sublingual application (under the tongue) and can be found in most health food stores.

STRESS.
We are told to meditate, take vacations, chill out or take calming drugs, but stress still takes its toll as a major contributor to illness. When the average person is under great stress for whatever reason, people compromise their eating habits. Instead of increasing the nutritious foods in their diet and adding necessary supplements, they eat fast foods, sugary snacks, and drink alcohol. These contribute to depression, fatigue, and aggravate their stressful condition. This also compromises their immune systems, making them more susceptible to illness, including the common cold. Sometimes the mental state becomes so aggravated, that they succumb to a diagnosis of mental illness. This can result in physicians prescribing an array of drugs.

Upon the recognition of the first stages of stress, we should improve our diets immediately. Besides the good basic food structure that most people are aware of, we need to supplement with certain nutrients that will improve our mental outlook. The immune system must be supported prior to treatment

135

for stress. Since the body has the ability to heal most of our ailments, we must give it the tools it needs to effect a cure. Adding extra minerals, enzymes and essential fatty acids to your diet gives your body the basics. Additionally, you can add specific herbs and other nutrients that reduce stress. Aged garlic extract has proven to actually reduce the effects of stress by lowering levels of corticoid, a hormone, which is secreted by the body during stress. This diminishes the effects stress has on our immune systems and our levels of energy. The primary effect stress has on our bodies is the toll it takes on our nervous system.

Stress depletes the brain's neurotransmitters. When faced with a stressful situation, the brain uses large amounts of feel-good transmitters, called endorphins. This upsets the ratio of many of the other transmitters, creating a chemical imbalance in the body. The result is increased anxiety and a sense of urgency. When psychological or sexual problems cause stressful situations, amino acid supplementation is necessary in order to avoid aggravating the neurotransmitter imbalance, and creating more stress. DL-phenylalanine and L-glutamine are key amino acids indicated in supporting neurotransmitter production that are keys to reducing stress.

Since the adrenal glands are negatively affected during times of stress, the following recommendations are listed. Licorice root has a specific use for adrenal support along with fresh wild oats, licorice Root, *Siberian Ginseng, *Fo-Ti extract. Eating adequate amounts of sea vegetables or taking kelp and cereal grass supplements will help support the adrenals. Stress relieving herbs that can reduce strain on the adrenals are hops, passionflower, skullcap and *ginseng.

Ginseng (Panax) has gained its reputation because of its ability to increase all-around well-being. As an adaptogenic (regulator) herb, ginseng helps the body deal with stress, increasing energy levels and decreasing fatigue. Another herb for stress reduction is valerian root. It is a strong, pain-relieving, safe sedative herb for anxiety, stress, PMS, menstrual cramping and emotional depression. It doesn't have the common side effects associated with narcotics used for similar purpose. It is an effective healer for the nervous system. Flower remedies may also assist in stress reduction when the emotions are involved. Aspen, dandelion, impatiens, lotus, sweet chestnut, vervain, chamomile and white chestnut flower combinations are used to clear mental strain and pressure, as well as relax muscles and calm the nervous system.

Following is a list of supplements that may help in stress reduction.
• Amino acid supplement
• Lecithin granules
• Liquid crystalloid electrolyte minerals
• Digestive enzymes taken with meals
• Flaxseed (ground)
• St. John's Wort and Ashwagandha herbs
• Kava-Kava herbal tinctures
• Multi-vitamin supplement
• Ginseng tea
• Calcium-magnesium supplement
• Flower remedies
• Additionally for men: Saw Palmetto extract or capsule
• Additionally for women: Don Quai extract
—Dosages vary depending on individuals, therefore we recommend consulting a health practitioner schooled in natural methods of preventive medicine.

VARICOSE VEINS.
This unsightly malady is the culmination of a low fiber, meat and dairy-based diet with too many refined foods. They also are indicated in vitamin E, C and A deficiencies, as well as from a lack of essential fatty acids. Pressure on the veins can stem from

excess weight (pregnancy included), as well as from chronic constipation. To reduce the acceleration of varicose veins, it is prudent to stick to good exercise program and to use an herbal massage compress over the affected area. Supplement your diet with bioflavonoids, aloe and wheatgrass. Drink three cups daily of white oak bark tea, and take garlic, MSM and vitamin E supplements. Hawthorne, butcher broom and gingko are good herbal remedies. To relieve the pain, bathe the legs in vinegar three times daily. Taking the cell salt Calc. Fluor. (Calcium Fluoride) will help to restore the elasticity to the vein, and cause contraction.

Recommended Reading.
•*Natural Solutions for Sexual Enhancement*, Dr. Howard Peiper &
Nina Anderson
Safe Goods Publishing
•*The Humorous Herbalist*, Laurel Dewey
Safe Goods Publishing
•*Left For Dead*, Dick Quinn
  Quinn Publishing
•*Healthy Healing*, Linda Rector Page
  Healthy Healing Publications
•*Excitotoxins: The Taste that Kills*. Dr. Russell Blaylock
  Health Press

THINK YOUNG

If you have been reading this book diligently and taking the information to heart, you might well be on the road to reversing the aging process by keeping a clean healthy body. In this chapter we will discuss the main tool to be used in creating a youthful you....the mind. How many times have people mentioned to you that *thoughts are things, be careful what you wish for, because you may get it (good and bad)* and *think positive*? Religions have taught that prayer will spawn miracles. Could it not be collective thought processes actually changing electrons, protons or whatever unseen molecule seems to make things happen? Christian Scientists have built a whole belief system on the power of the mind and they have produced some pretty remarkable results.

A friend, general manager of a major sports team, burned himself horribly when a gas grill flared up in his face. Rather than seek medical help and an arduous recovery, which included skin grafting, he left his fate to Christian Scientist friends who kept him in a bedroom, sight unseen, for a week. Outside this room they visualized his face as being perfectly recovered, and without pain. They instructed the "patient" to do the same. With very minimal topical applications of some herbal salve and with very strong mind techniques, this man fully recovered without medical help, and today has no scars or trace of his accident.

The medical profession is now acknowledging the power of the mind to heal. The government of the USA just admitted to including psychics on their payroll, for espionage purposes. A new medical term 'subtle energies', has recently been invented to describe the effects the mind has on influencing the body, and an organization has been formed around that theory, the International Society for the Study of Subtle Energies and Energy Medicine (ISSSEEM). Mind control is not new news, it's just coming out of the closet. In the following pages, we will mostly discuss how the mind affects the body's ability to make itself sick or well, but if you carry this further, you will see how your thoughts determine whether you become old as you age, or stay young.

Since the baby boomers are all arriving at that magic age where retirement is starting to become a reality, corporate America is responding with media coverage targeting the 'older' person. Nursing homes and retirement communities are advertising on TV, and many of them focus on the elderly as being needy, gray, hunched over beings no longer wishing to be a burden on their children. If this is what is implanted in the mind over and over again, what do you think will surface? Expectations beget reality, and if you are prone to think that you will shrink and get hunched over by the time you are 70, then you will. On the other hand...like one TV ad shows, you could be in your 70s, and still jumping hurdles in a track competition. It's up to you!

This chapter is written in collaboration with Dr. William Lowe Mundy, M.D., a personal friend and currently Clinical Professor of Medicine at the University of Missouri School of Medicine in Kansas City. He maintains a private practice specializing in Psychosomatic Disease, Internal Medicine and Psychotherapy and has written a book about his techniques for visual imagery. Through clinical observations, experiments and personal experiences, Dr. Mundy has broadened his approach to healing to include alternative treatments, and recognizes the power of the mind to influence the body's ability to heal or hurt itself. If we follow his techniques, we may just be able to turn back our biological clock psychologically. The following text is excerpted from his writings and lectures.

"In the last couple of decades we have seen some startling results from research done in a field called psychoneuro-immunology. It is wonderful to think that we can actually voluntarily change our immune system, once thought to be autonomic and not in our control, by utilizing specific kinds of thought patterns.

A group of volunteers can have regular blood counts done at the start of an experiment and the number and kind of white blood cells determined. Shown a slide of white blood cells, they then utilize simple relaxation techniques and for a quiet hour are asked to imagine that they are increasing the number of those cells. At the end of the hour, their blood counts are again determined. There is a highly significant increase in cells. It is even possible to increase not just the total number of white blood cells, but to increase a specific kind.

This imagery is the mind's way of reminding you of the way something looked, sounded, felt, smelled or tasted. We use imagery all the time. If I decide to scratch myself where I itch, I must, of necessity, process the location of the discomfort and then 'image' my finger to go to that place. I have to be in control of that motion from the very inception of the thought of wanting to scratch. In milliseconds, I imagine with my mind's eye how my finger will go to the place I have chosen, and it does!

I used to think of the body as being comprised of different organs, all working together, and each having their own special set of cells. This in itself seemed pretty miraculous. What in the world could have been the mediator, who could be the manager, who or what could possibly coordinate all these happenings that make us operate?

Some doctor friends believe these accomplishments are due in some miraculous fashion to a proper mingling of chemicals in the brain that somehow are able to send messages down pathways called motor nerves, those connected serially, one to the next, with spaces called synapses. Each message would have to go through a series of chemical transactions in order to get to the end organ, and then have the success of the movement transmitted back to the brain by another set of nerves, called sensory. I can't imagine how a bunch of chemicals can initiate a thought, a desire to move, and be able to choose just which connecting links are needed to effect the desire.

Think of a really complicated process, like playing the piano. Can you possibly imagine that ten fingers, moving all at once and with amazing deliberate direction, and combined with a foot pedal working along with them. The fingers are motivated in some way through the interpretation of the visual perception processed by the mind, off the pages of a musical score, and listened to by an auditory mechanism in such a finite way that the hands can place less or more energy to the keys. This is all dependent on the congruency of the comfort level of the performer, changing speed, tone and timbre at will, and even remotely believing that such amazing coordination could be under the control of a bunch of chemicals??!!

A group of patients suffering from cancer are instructed to construct in their mind a cartoon-like picture of their own cancer cells, and again image a picture of what they think their immune cells can do to eradicate the cancer cells. They then practice this little play in their mind for an extended period of time, and sure enough, it is found that these patients do far better in ameliorating, and sometimes curing their cancers than the non-imagers. Are those results due to a set of chemicals?

What we know as a placebo effect is now accepted as real by the medical profession. What amazing things must have happened between mind and body to explain how someone is given a prescription (placebo) by Great Father Doctor, believing it would be of benefit, and sure enough, they got well? To think that we never stopped to investigate why a placebo worked!

How you think (processing pieces of information) results in how you feel (the emotions you have following your thinking), and ends up causing a change in the body. For instance something goes wrong (you think), and you get so 'up tight' (emotion) that your blood pressure rises (physical manifestation). Emotional reactions of all sorts create bodily

142

responses of organs not connected by nerve pathways. Continued stress somehow alerts the adrenals to produce more steroids, the liver to start producing more glycogen, the spleen to get more cells into action; all miraculously working together to preserve our wellness.

Most of us have simply accepted that our body's responses to our emotions are automatic, and yet we have all experienced a time when we taught ourselves to defy these emotions, and got a different result. We have the power, the capacity, to feel miserable as, well as happy. For most of us, it is easy to 'image' a person and circumstances to have what is called a sexual fantasy. We can utilize a goal-oriented scheme in our mind to change the function of our body, by imaging the parts we wish to contact, and sending those parts a message.

All too often doctors are prone to believe that emotional problems, such as depression, occur as a result of disease. I believe that emotions can also cause a disease. Most people don't realize that they learned a long time ago to have the depression they suffer with today. Whatever you were taught, whatever learnings you incorporated as a child, can be unlearned. If one feels helpless and victimized by fate and their own sense of inadequacy, the immune system would be hard put to be of much help with visual imagery; therefore, these feelings and the resultant depression must be resolved before visual imagery can work. Several years ago, I met two women who had Lupus Erythematosis, and who became aware of the relationship of their depression and their disease. With devoted effort, they not only cured their depression, they stopped having the disease.

I have been successful ridding people of their allergies by visual imagery. Somewhere along the line our immune systems decided the good guys (tourists) were bad guys (terrorists) and decided to fight them...thus, a la, allergies. Through simple imagery, we can re-educate the immune system to embrace the tourists, and not confuse them with the terrorists, thereby getting

143

rid of our allergic reactions. If you don't believe some allergies are created in the mind, explain why many allergic people sneeze at pictures of flowers, when there is absolutely no pollen around.

Quality of life is important to maintain as we age, and we all want health, happiness (and money) in our later years. Goal-setting and taking an Anthony Robbins course may get you the money and some happiness, but you have to create your own good health. According to the relevant literature, psychological factors may play an important role in the onset and clinical course of rheumatoid arthritis, a common ailment in older persons. Studies have shown that joint tenderness from arthritis is more prevalent in patients with lower levels of self-esteem.

Unhappy emotions and poor self-image can lead to disease. In one study on patients with multiple sclerosis, 28 of the 32 people interviewed revealed that their transition into MS coincided with a psychologically stressful situation, one which mobilized feelings of helplessness. Since multiple sclerosis is commonly thought to be related at least in part to alterations in the immune system, it is possible to speculate that immune mechanisms, which are already compromised, can undergo further destabilization under some circumstances, in the face of severe or chronic emotional upset. "Does this mean we play a part in creating disease?"

I am sure there are many patients, along with their doctors, who are unwilling to believe that they can be a part of their own cure. They may be unwilling to deal with their own emotional states, and would be loathe to undertake a therapeutic approach, in which they would have to stop viewing themselves as victims, and would be asked to take an aggressive role in their healing. Visual imagery is a completely normal and necessary process used by every person every day. All we are doing, with a more therapeutic process, is to design a goal-oriented method of contacting parts of the body that we here to fore have considered unavailable. Visual imagery makes it possible for us to take part in our own health and well-being. It is easy to do and completely harmless. The power of the mind can be curative. Using new thoughts, creating re-perceptions and imaging in innovative ways, as we re-frame, healing can be done within the mind without verbalization or conversation with a therapist.

As people age, they seem to accept that their bodies are bound to deteriorate, and that they are at risk for debilitating illness. By practicing imagery, as described in the book, *Curing Allergy with Visual Imagery*, you can change that thought, and create for yourself a different consequence. In using imagery to cure allergies, I ask my patients to think of themselves as Disney cartoonists. Getting away from realism is easier for most people to do. It relieves them of the need to be perfect, and makes the imaging a fun kind of thing. We know that the information is understood by the cells, no matter how incongruous someone's idea of what magnified elements might look like. It is the ideas behind the imagery plot that we want to get across, and accuracy of method doesn't seem to be significant. Perhaps the immune system likes a happier, yet effective way of going about the job."

If you are not willing to accept this concept of the way our mind, body and spirit work together and of the mind being present in all of our parts, then explain in your own way how the outcome of imagery, when used to change cellular function, definitely works. I can find no other way to explain such marvelous happenings. And think of it this way, to quote Richard Bach, Not knowing doesn't keep the truth from being true. Remember, you are what you think.

Recommended reading:
•*Curing Allergy With Visual Imagery*, Dr. Wm. Lowe Mundy
  Available through ATN Group (888) 217-7233

FITNESS FOR YOUTH

Beginning a fitness program can be as easy as taking a walk every day. Walking is a natural movement for the body, and helps to strengthen bone and muscle, as it exercises the heart and lungs. As we age, even as early as 35, we begin to lose muscle mass and about 1% of bone mass per year. For post menopausal women, the percentage may as much as quadruple. Beginning an exercise program that includes weight bearing exercises such as walking, cycling and running, can not only increase your muscle and bone mass, but decrease your body fat as well. Walking at a pace that elevates your heart rate is considered an aerobic activity. This exercises the heart and lungs, and this puts you at a lower risk level for diabetes, heart disease, hypertension, and osteoporosis.
—*It's always a good idea to check with your physician before beginning any exercise program.*

To get on your way to feeling wonderfully fit and healthy, start your walking program today! You'll need a good pair of walking shoes and comfortable clothes. Layering is always a good idea. A good way to get in tune with your body is by feeling how hard you are working. Familiarize yourself with your perceived exertion level. Zero is standing still and ten is when you are almost out of breath. You should strive for a level of 6 to 8 which means you should be able to carry on a conversation without becoming breathless. If this is happening to you, slow your pace down a bit. Strive for 60-70%.

AGE	MAX. HEART RATE	60%	70%
30	195	115	133
40	180	110	126
50	170	105	119
60	160	95	112
70	150	85	105
80	140	75	98

To begin your program, you should walk at a comfortable pace for about five minutes, stop and stretch your calves, hamstrings, and quadriceps, holding each stretch for about twenty seconds. The reason for walking before you stretch is to warm up the muscles. Stretching cold muscles can lead to injury so be sure to walk first, then stretch.

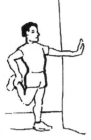 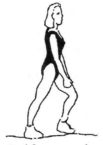 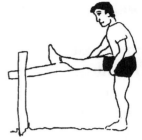

Quad stretch   Calf stretch   Hamstring stretch

Select a program that is right for you from the following: Beginner level: walk for 15-20 minutes, 3 times/week. Intermediate: walk for 25-45 minutes, 4-5 times/week. Advanced: walk for 45-60 minutes, 5-7 times/week. If you're a beginner, stay with the first program until you find it too easy, and increase your time gradually. Also, remember to drink plenty of water. Staying hydrated when you exercise is very important, especially in hot weather.

A fun way to increase your endurance and put variety in you work out is to use "fartlek", a Swedish word meaning speedplay. During your walk, look for mailboxes, telephone poles, driveways, etc., and increase your speed from one to the next. For example, after you've walked for about ten minutes, walk fast from one driveway to the next, then resume your normal pace. Do this up to ten times during your walk. Once this becomes easy, try increasing your pace for two driveways, then three, etc. It's fun and it helps you to stay motivated.

If you want to try something more challenging, and your physician tells you it's OK to run, try walking for two minutes, then jog or run for one. (of course, this is after you've warmed up and stretched). Another challenge is to switch your walking time to one minute, and run for two, or walk two and run two. There are lots of ways to keep from getting bored. The main objective is to have fun, and enjoy what you're doing.

If possible, try to vary your course, or walk up hills to challenge your body. Variety wards off boredom, so try to change the scenery, or walk with a friend to keep things interesting. If you find yourself short on time, a ten minute walk can do wonders for you mentally, and any time spent exercising is better than none at all. When you've completed your walk, be sure to stretch the same muscles you did after your warm up. This will prevent soreness and help to keep you injury free.

An important component of exercise for those over fifty is strength training. For each decade of life, adults lose approximately six pounds of muscle. Muscle strength decreases by about twenty percent by age sixty-five, along with a decrease in flexibility. Regular strength training not only prevents some of this loss, but increases bone and muscle mass and flexibility. Studies have shown that a regular strength-training program can add about three pounds of muscle mass in approximately two months. Researchers in Gainsville, Florida had men and women, ranging in age from sixty to eighty-two, exercise for six months, using special back-strengthening machines. The results showed that their spinal bone density increased by fourteen percent. This is especially significant for women, because they lose ten to fifteen percent of the minerals needed to sustain bone in their spines during the ten years following menopause.

Strength training for women and men over fifty is critical to staying active in later years. Bones need to be subjected to stress in order to increase density and generate bone growth. Lifting weights provides the stress needed to do this, while muscles, tendons, and ligaments become stronger. Your sense of balance is improved, along with reaction time, both of which help prevent falls. Fractured hips and spines are all too common occurrences in those over 65, and a basic strength training program can help prevent this. Beginning now can help you look and feel great, plus help keep you healthy and strong for years to come!

Many of us have a problem with weight gain as we get older, and although aerobic exercise is one way to lose weight, research has shown that a combination of aerobics and strength training is the best way to reduce body fat. Although you may expend more calories during aerobic activities, the rate at which you burn calories (metabolic rate) remains elevated for a longer period of time following strength training. Your body expends thirty to fifty calories just maintaining the muscle you are building!

To begin a strength training program, you'll want to plan on working out two to three times per week. It's important to wait at least twenty four hours before working the same muscles again. Muscles need adequate time to recover and rebuild. The following program is designed to work major muscle groups in approximately twenty to thirty minutes, however, if you want to increase your strength, you can simply do two to three sets instead of one. The American College of Sports Medicine recommends eight to ten exercises for major muscle groups, eight to twelve repetitions with a minimum of one set, and exercising a minimum of two times per week.

— *Again, always check with your physician before starting an exercise program.*

Be sure to warm up your muscles first with some sort of rhythmic limbering by walking, marching in place, walking on a treadmill, using a stationary bike, dancing to music...whatever you like to do for five to ten minutes. Follow this with static stretches for the major muscle groups. Hold each stretch for at least twenty seconds, and be careful not to bounce! Begin with

large muscle groups and progress to smaller muscles for a safe, well- rounded program.
Additional Stretches:

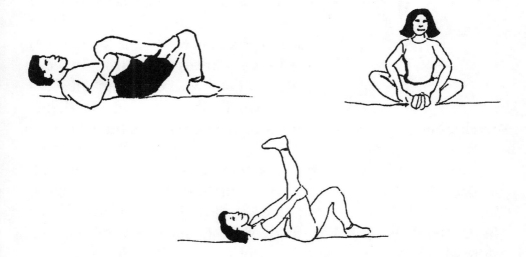

After you have warmed up, begin each exercise slowly, taking one to two seconds for each movement, exhaling with exertion.

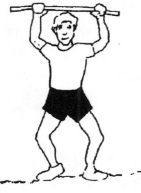

1. Stand with your knees unlocked, feet should be a shoulder width apart and toes pointed out. Hold a resistance band (like a giant flat rubber band), in your hands and lift both hands over-head, pulling out, creating resistance against the bands. Keeping abdominals contracted, pull arms down and back while you do a slight knee bend. Return to beginning position. Do 8-12 repetitions. This works the back (latissimus dorsi) and lower body.

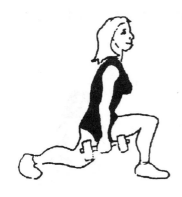

2. With your hands on your hips, or at your sides, holding 1-3 lb. weights, lunge forward with the right leg. Modify this exercise by making a small lunge (or lunge backward if you have a problem with your knees). Do not let your knees go in front of your toes. Do 8-12 with each leg. This exercise works the front of the thighs (quadriceps), back of leg (hamstrings) and buttocks (gluteals).

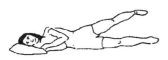

3. Lie on your side, with legs extended, and your head resting on your forearm, the other hand on floor in front of your chest. You may use 1-3 lb. ankle weights. Flex foot and lift your leg to about hip level, being careful not to roll back. Lower the leg back to floor. Do 8-10 repetitions then repeat with the other leg. This works the outer thigh muscles (abductors).

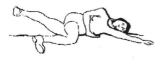

4. Stay on your side and drop the top leg in front of you on the floor. Lift the back leg up to work the inner thigh muscles. return it to the floor. Do this 8-10 times, and repeat with the other leg, being careful not to roll back. The most effective way to do this exercise is slowly, pausing for a moment at the top. Works the hip adductors.

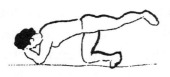

5. On "all fours", with ankle weights, resistance bands or nothing at all, with abdominals contracted, keeping your back flat, rest on your forearms, keeping your knees under your hips; lift and straighten one leg, then slowly bend the knee so that your heel curls toward the buttocks. Straighten the leg. Do 8-12 before repeating with other

leg. Be careful not to arch your back. This works the back of the leg (hamstrings).

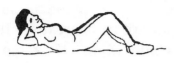

6A. Lay on your back with your knees bent, and your hands across your chest or behind the head with elbows out. Think of having an orange under your chin to prevent you from pushing your chin onto your chest as you raise. Tighten abdominals and lift your shoulders off floor, while bringing a knee toward your chest. Do 10 - 30 repetitions, alternating legs. Exhale as you lift up. This works the upper and lower muscles of the abdominals.

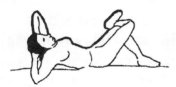

6B. To work the obliques (waist muscles) , stay on your back with your knees bent, and cross the right ankle over the left knee. With your hands behind your head, keep the right elbow on floor and lift diagonally while exhaling, bringing the left shoulder (not elbow) toward the knee. Return to the floor. Do 8-15 repetitions on each side.

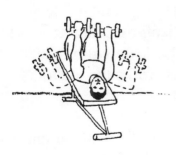

7. Stay on your back with your knees bent and abdominals contracted. Hold resistance bands or 1-3 lb. weights in both hands, and raise your arms towards the ceiling with your hands almost touching. Move your arms out and down until your elbows touch the floor, exhaling as you go. Slowly bring the arms back up to your beginning position. Do 8-12 repetitions.
This works the chest (pectoralis muscles).

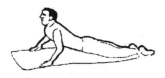

8. In a face down position, contract the lower back muscles and lift the chest off the floor, using the arms slightly to assist you. Hold for a moment, and then return to starting position. Be careful not to overextend the lower back, or to throw the head back while lifting. Do 8 repetitions (reps). This works the low back.

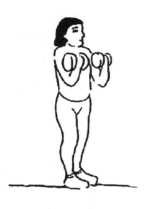

9. Stand up, with your feet a hip width apart, abdominals contracted, and your arms at your sides, palms up. Hold 1-3 lb. weight in each hand, if desired. Keeping elbows tight against sides, curl your hands up to your shoulders, exhaling as you lift, then slowly lower to starting position. Don't swing weights. Do 8-12 reps. This works the biceps.

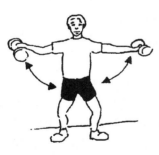

10. Remaining in the same position, and holding 1-3 lb. weights at your sides, palms in, lift your arms out to your sides just to shoulder level, elbows slightly bent, exhaling as you lift. Slowly lower back down to sides. Do 8-12 reps. This works the deltoids (shoulders).

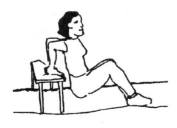

11. To do triceps dips, sit on an armless chair, with your hands holding the front of the seat, with fingers pointing down. Move forward until your hips come off the chair, and lower buttocks to the floor. Press up with your arms

for full extension, arms straight, but not locked. Keep feet firmly on the floor with knees bent. Repeat 8 -12 times.
This works the back of arms (triceps).

To complete your strength training program, it's important to finish by stretching the muscles you've just worked. This will prevent soreness, help to resume normal resting length of the muscle and increase flexibility. You should enjoy your time spent stretching. Repeat the stretches given at the beginning of this chapter, holding each for at least twenty to thirty seconds.

Relaxation is a wonderful bonus to add to your workout when you have time. You'll find it relieves tension and stress and gives you renewed energy. Find a quiet spot or play some relaxing music. Think of your mind as a blackboard, and erase all writing on the board to clear you mind. Imagine yourself in a place that you love, perhaps the beach, hearing the waves gently rolling to shore, feeling the warmth of the sun on your body. Take deep, diaphragmatic breaths (belly breathing), and exhale very slowly. Try to think of the peaceful sensation you are feeling as a color, bathing you slowly from head to toe. Beginning at your feet, relax muscle by muscle, pausing at each one to enjoy the feeling. Continue to breathe deeply and slowly. When you feel completely relaxed, think of something that makes you happy, that makes you smile. Bring it to the front of your mind and keep it there until the next time you do this exercise. Staying active can help us live our lives to their fullest.

Appendix.

Nutritional supplement selection. Regarding the selection of nutritional supplements, there have been some extraordinary advances made. Humans have been successful in obtaining the nutrients we need to sustain life for as long as we have inhabited the planet. It is only since the 1920's that we have been adding dietary supplements that are synthesized in a laboratory.

Ingesting vitamin and mineral supplements in this processed form only delivers a fraction of the whole food. These are considered fractionalized nutrients. The human body is designed to obtain our nutrients from food which contains the naturally occurring vital food co-factors. This is a simple but important issue. When nutrients are *isolated* and put into tablet form, we are circumventing nature's natural pathways and going against "Mother Nature."

Food is so complex that scientists are unable to map its exact structure. As an example, a tomato contains over 10,000 vitamins, minerals and other phyto-nutrients. Food sustains life, but fractions of nutrients from food do not accomplish this satisfactorily. We need the complete package to create synergy in the body, not just a part. Most companies and therefore, most consumers believe that ascorbic acid is vitamin C. This is not the case. Studies have shown that when 100% pure ascorbic acid is given to scurvy patients, it doesn't work as well as vitamin C from food sources. This is because the 100% ascorbic acid does not contain the co-factors necessary for proper assimilation. When nutrients are synthesized, they no longer possess the qualities of whole food. The extremely important vital food co-factors are missing.

There have been some truly exciting technological advances made in recent years that allow us to ingest nutrients in a concentrated whole food form. New processes allow us to connect the vital food factors with the nutrients in food cells. Taking whole food supplements gives you nutrients in a complex form with the co-factors in tact. These co-factors may be carbohydrates, proteins, phyto-nutrients and thousands of other components which comprise food. They create advanced absorption and utilization through a natural delivery system, not found in ordinary vitamin and mineral supplements. Supplements that are not absorbed are not used by the body, and when they are excreted, become very expensive toilet water.

Therefore, when selecting supplements, remember there are distinctly different forms of nutrients. All forms of nutrients have value. The body responds to these forms of nutrients in uniquely different ways. We know that all vitamin C supplements are not alike, and the same principle applies to minerals, vitamins, herbs and other immune-support products. We as consumers, must educate ourselves. Just as we read labels to avoid preservatives and additives on packaged foods, we must be discriminating about our supplement purchases.

RESOURCE DIRECTORY

TACHYONIZED™ WATER. Proven to be a valuable ingredient for maintaining radiant health, high energy and addressing imbalanced conditions, these drops, taken sublingually breaks the blood-brain barrier and instantly provides life force energy to the body. *Tachyonized™ Silica Gel* can strengthen skin, hair, bones, nails, ligaments and tendons. *Tachyonized™ Fizz-C* provides the body with 2 gm. vitamin C and 7 minerals, all Tachyonized™ to magnify and accelerate their effects on the body's absorption and energy utilization. ADVANCED TACHYON TECHNOLOGIES, 480 Tesconi Ci., Santa Rosa, CA 95401 (800) 966-9341   www.tachyon-energy.com

NATURALLY ALOE JUICE PRODUCTS. Aloe Commodities processes and packages high quality aloe vera beverages. The products are made with organically grown aloe vera plants and are certified by the International Aloe Science Council for purity and content. Aloe Commodities was recognized for quality products by receiving the 1998 "Peoples choice" award, at the NNFA convention in the category of nutritional drinks. ALOE COMMODITIES INTERNATIONAL, INC., 12901 Nicholson 370, Farmers Branch TX 75234 (800) 701-2563

ALL NATURAL TOXIN REMOVAL. ARISE & SHINE'S *Cleanse Thyself Program™*, as developed by Dr. Richard Anderson, N.D., N.M.D., is the most effective all-natural way of removing toxins and unwanted waste materials from the body today. These toxins build up in layers in the colon and intestines and prevent the body from properly absorbing vitamins and health supplements. Commonly reported benefits from The *Cleanse Thyself* detoxification program are: improved health, more energy, greater clarity of mind, improved stamina, better skin tone and improved physiological function. Free catalogue/information packet available. ARISE & SHINE HERBAL PRODUCTS, P.O. Box 1439, Mt. Shasta, CA 96067 (800) 688-2444

CHLOROPHYLL PRODUCTS: DeSouza's Liquid Chlorophyll is a versatile product that can be taken as a dietary supplement or used as a mouthwash and breath freshener. It contains no preservatives or flavorings and come in capsules or tablets. The newly formulated *TOOTH GEL* is a breakthrough homeopathic dental care product that includes baking soda for whiter cleaner teeth and potentized Cats Claw that is known for its positive effects on the gums. *TOOTH GEL* is free from sodium lauryl sulfphate and contains legendary alfalfa-derived sodium copper chlorophyllin, an excellent breath freshener. Also available is *DeSouza's ORAL RINSE and SPRAY*, an excellent cleansing agent, astringent and breath freshener with natural cinnamon flavor. Only the purest of water is used, with Ascorbic Acid added as a preservative and it is alcohol free. *DeSouza's HAND and BODY LOTION* now contains Vitamin C which cleanses moisturizes and beautifies the skin. With this fragrance-free reformulated product both men and women will enjoy healthy, youthful looking skin. DeSOUZA INTERNATIONAL, INC., PO Box 395, Beaumont, CA 92223 (800) 373-5171
www.desouzas.com

REVERSE DIMINISHING MEMORY. *MemorEase*™ formulation is backed by two randomized placebo-controlled clinical studies. *MemorEase*™ (1) can reverse the effects of aging on memory function in healthy adults, (2) block the progression of senile dementia in diagnosed individuals, and (3) block the onset of "winter blues" depression. *MemorEase*™ is a proprietary blend of oxidation stable phosphatidyl serine (PS) and cell metabolism stimulating phosphatidic acid (PA). *MemorEase*™ is all-natural and contains no animal by-products or hexane chemical residue. Also available, *Seasilver,* which contains organic sea vegetables, Aloe vera and Pau D'arco. *Seasilver* provides in nature's perfect balance at the cellular level , every vitamin, macro-mineral, trace mineral, amino acid and enzyme known to man. Some of the benefits are: purifies the blood, cleanses the vital organs, nourishes the body, oxygenates at a cellular level and strengthens the immune system. Ajit Channe, President, G.K. PRODUCTS, INC. 10088 N.W. 3rd Place, Coral Springs, FL 33071 (888) 752-4286

POWERFUL HEALING TEA. *EZZEAC PLUS*™ *ORIGINAL and EZZEAC Plus CAT'S CLAW* have three times the herbs used by other brands. The first is the original formula from the Ojibway Indians. Unlike all other brands, some of the herbs in this formula are never boiled therefore the live enzymes are not destroyed. They also contain the correct amount of watercress as an ingredient to help protect the kidneys. *EZZEAC PLUS*™ *Teas* may be used to help detoxify the blood, kidney and the liver and has been historically used in cases of chronic disease. CAT'S CLAW herb stimulates the immune system and kills pathogens. Phytochemicals have powerful anti-microbial, anti-ulcer, anti-inflammatory, anti-allergic, anti-oxidant, anti-tumor and it also contains adaptogen properties. GREEN LEAF HERBS (800) 770-1080

FRESH FROM THE FARM. FLAX FOR YOUR IMMUNE SYSTEM. A whole food, *Dakota Flax Gold* is all natural edible fresh flax seed, is high in lignins which can be used over cereal, on salads, in soups or in juice. Ready to grind, just like your best coffee, it is low in cadmium and is better tasting than packaged flax products. Seeds must be ground for full nutritional value. Dakota Flax Gold is available with grinder. Flax, and also available in capsule form as *Flaxeon Jet,* is a convenient way of getting beneficial essential fatty acids. Another product, *DiaBran* is made from 100% Pure RiceX Stabilized Rice Bran which contains as close as possible, all the nutrients created by nature that the body needs to maintain health. Taking *DiaBran* can increase energy levels, blood glucose balance and prevent some illness. HEINTZMAN FARMS, RR2 Box 265, Onaka SD 57466   (800) 333-5813   (send S.A.S.E. for sample)
                                                                www.heintzmanfarms.com

BLUE GREEN ALGAE, ONE OF EARTH'S MOST COMPLETE FOODS. One of the main keys for staying young and vibrant is *Blue Green Algae*. Millions use *Blue Green Algae* for everything from better energy, increased stamina, increased virility, increased T-cells, to beautify skin as well as reports of weight reduction. Order from an expert in the field with over fourteen years direct experience with *Blue Green Algae*. KBC INC. (727) 446-0819 *pH TESTING PAPERS: pH Hydrion* Papers test the acid/alkaline condition of your urine. With readings of 5.5 to 8.0, these strips can indicate balance in the body and determine which food to eat to rebalance your system. LONG LIFE CATALOG CO., P.O. Box 968., Nokomis, FL. 34274 (888) NATURE-1

ALL NATURAL ALTERNATIVE FOR IMPOTENCY. CholestoPlex and *CardioPlex* offer nutritional support for healthy cholesterol levels and a healthy strong heart which are important factors for a satisfying sex life. Also for sexual support, *RexHard* is a blend of essential nutrients, vitamins, minerals and amino acids combined with potent herbal extracts. *RexHard* improves desire, performance and firmness for increased sexual pleasure. It increases energy and circulation. MAMAR LABS, INC., 4646 Domestic Ave. #101, Naples FL 34104   (800) 862-3931
Email: mamar33@aol.com   www.mamar-labs.com

VELVET ANTLER CAPSULES. Historically, Ve*lvet antler* has been used for more than 2,000 years in several cultures around the world. Since velvet antler is said to build up the body's natural resources, many consider it one of the most versatile all around health food supplements, and is becoming known as nature's perfect food. During antler growth high levels of natural hormones are present in the blood, including IGF-1 and II which plays an important role in growth and development. New studies in North America have identified the velvet of elk antlers as containing collagen as a major protein, rich in glycosaminoglycans (GAGs). Chondroitin sulfate is the major GAG in antler. The elk are raised on farms in North America and the velvet antler harvested annually without causing harm to the animal. It is processed and then encapsulated at a FDA inspected laboratory. MEADOW CREEK ELK FARMS, 7860 Woodland Lane, West Bend, WI 53090 (800) 547-8450 #01   www.hnet.net/~elkacres

WHOLE FOOD CONCENTRATES IN SUPPLEMENT FORM: As food, FoodState® nutrients are delivered with a matrix of Vital food Factors™ such as carbohydrates, proteins, phyto-nutrients and the thousands of other components which comprise food. These vital food factors™ create advanced absorption and utilization through a natural delivery system called Protein Chaperones™. This superior delivery system is not found in ordinary vitamins and minerals. Absorption, utilization, efficacy and safety are all primary concerns when creating *MegaFod™ DailyFoods™* formulas. All *MegaFood™* formulas exclusively use 100% FoodState® nutrients to ensure these concerns are addressed. *MegaFood™* FoodState® nutrients are hydroponically farmed (Nutrient Activation or Grown in water). These processes require meticulous care. Scientific instrumentation is crucial. Samples of the FoodState® nutrients are tested at regular intervals in a state of the art, FDA registered laboratory to determine the exact time when the Growth and Activation processes are complete. Only at this point, when the FoodState® nutrients test perfect, are they harvested. This extensive testing enables *MegaFood™* to assure that you are receiving the most bountiful source of nutrients, 100% complex food. Available in 23 tableted formulas. MEGA FOODS., 8 Bowers Road., Derry NH 03038 (800) 258-5014 *For more details on FoodState® nutrients see nutritional supplement selection appendix.*

ANTI-AGING FLOWER REMEDIES. Flower remedies treat the emotional side of illness and are effective in reducing symptoms of illness that stem from our inner thoughts. *Fearfulness* is excellent to relieve menopausal panic attacks. *Stress/Tension* clears mental strain and pressure, relaxes tense muscles and calms and strengthens the nervous system. *Forgetfulness* assists with memory lapses and loss, wandering thoughts, lack of alertness and attentiveness, senility and amnesia. *Worry/Concern* is for those who are concerned about aging and death. NATURAL LABS CORP., P.O. Box 20037, Sedona AZ 86341-0037 (800) 233-0810

LIQUID CRYSTALLOID MINERALS AND CAL/MAG SUPPLEMENT: Minerals: *Trace-Lyte™* is a true crystalloid (smallest form in nature) electrolyte formula that helps maintain the body's primary bio-oxidation process. It raises the Osmotic Pressure of the cell walls, strengthening them! It changes back the pH of the cell to its healthy state. This process is generally referred to as homeostasis (electrolyte balance). High absorption is achieved due to its crystalloid structure. Some doctors have even said it acts like 'chelation' in a bottle! Unlike most earth-type liquid minerals, there is no heavy metal contaminates whatsoever. Calcium/magnesium supplement: Many health authorities have recently stated that osteoporosis is reaching epidemic proportions in our country! This appears to be happening to men as well as women. Recently, research has shown that by supplementing our diets with good quality 1 to 1 ratio of calcium and magnesium, we may not only stop the thinning of our bones, but in fact, rebuild them! *Cal-Lyte™* with electrolytes and boron can give you this assurance and its super absorption formula can reduce muscle soreness, all forms of cramping and low back pain. NATURE'S PATH, INC. PO Box 7862, Venice FL 34287-7862 (800) 326-5772, (941) 426-3375 fax (941) 426-6871

HERBAL/MINERAL SKIN SPRAY: *Skin-Lyte™* is a perfect blend of the best nature has to offer. It encourages rapid absorption of vital mineral nutrients to aid in skin rejuvenation, and is combined with a blend of ancient herbal extracts to help in healing. *Skin-Lyte™* is a fusion of crystalloid electrolyte minerals ionically bound with herbal extracts in a base of pure water. Water carries away nutrient, contributes to normal tissue structure, lubricates and flushes away toxins. With consistent use, *Skin-Lyte's™* herbs and crystalloid minerals balance pH and provide intense, deep nourishment to the skin aiding healing and rejuvenation. NATURE'S PATH, INC. PO Box 7862, Venice, FL 34287-7862 (800) 326-5772

YOUTH THROUGH ELECTROLYTES. *Total-Lyte* is a 70% protein cracked cell yeast that has been shown to increase mental efficiency, improve concentration, nourish the brain and combat fatigue. It is an essential part in keeping the mind and body healthy. *Bio-Lyte* contains bioflavonoids that prevent arteries from hardening and enhance blood vessels, capillary and vein strength. It also lowers cholesterol and stimulate bile production. *Leci-Lyte* is a unique blend of lecithin and crystalloid electrolytes. It is one of nature's perfect brain foods, helping to ward off the mental diseases of old age. NATURE'S PATH, INC. PO Box 7862, Venice, FL 34287-7862 (800) 326-5772

HEIGHTEN SEXUAL PROWESS. Finally, a natural health product that delivers what it promises. This supplement will do more for the male libido than any other. *Amoré-Lyte* actually can restore the libido to its fullest capacity. And, there are NO side effects!! This is truly a totally natural formula that works. Another fantastic feature of this unique product is the addition of crystalloid electrolytes, which both act as a synergistic factor for the libido and, through a process known as biovection, the electrolytes act as a super carrier of the nutrients to the body's cells. *Amoré-Lyte* helps to maintain a healthy 'toning' of the prostate gland so important today. Also available is *Pollen-Lyte.* Among its many properties, bee pollen has the ability to help maintain the integrity of the cell, and foster immune support. Plus, in years past, bee pollen has shown great power in restoring body functioning including the rebuilding of the reproductive system. *Pollen-Lyte* provides bee pollen together with crystalloid electrolytes for maximum utilization in the body. NATURE'S PATH, INC. PO Box 7862, Venice, FL 34287-7862   (800) 326-5772

JUMP START YOUR HEALTH. TRI-HOMEOPATHIC SYSTEM. This kit contains three of the most vital homeopathic formulations for health restoration and/or health maintenance. The *#1 Detoxifier,* taken every day before bedtime, helps the body to remove metabolic and environmental toxins. The *#29 Bowel Discomfort,* taken before meals, helps to relieve intestinal symptoms and promote good digestion. *The #9 Rheumatic Pain,* taken daily, helps relieve pain symptoms and assists the body in the removal of uric acid, a potentially harmful free radical. NEWTON LABORATORIES, 2360 Rockaway Industrial Blvd., Conyers, GA 30012 (800) 448-7256 Email:mailinfo@newtonlabs.net   www.newtonlabs.net

100% VEGETARIAN ENZYMES: *Nutri-Essence™ Broad Spectrum Enzymes™* help maximize food nutrient value by replacing the enzymes destroyed when food is cooked or processed. These enzymes are 100% vegetarian and are available in VEGICAPS® or great-tasting raspberry chewable tablets. NUTRI-ESSENCE™ DIV. OF ENZYMES, INC., 8500 NW River Park Dr., Parkville, MO 64152 (800) 647-6377 Fax (800) 844-1957

NATURAL ANSWER TO THE DECLINING HORMONE LEVELS OF MIDLIFE. Nutrition Now® announces an addition to its popular line of women's products: *Menopause Complete™.* Each box contains two powerful products that work together to support women who are experiencing menopause. *Menopause Plus™* capsules include all-natural vitamins, traditional herbs and soy isoflavones for strong nutritional support. *Pro-Estro™* cream with Mexican wild yam, a natural progesterone, is a greaseless and odorless cream that is absorbed through the skin for time-sustained effectiveness. The *Menopause Complete™* team is a complete, natural answer to the declining hormone levels of midlife. Staying healthy is not easy in this day and age. Busy lifestyles, prescription drugs and hormonal changes often lead to digestive troubles, fatigue and yeast infections. *PB 8® Pro-Biotic Acidophilus* helps keep your system in tip-top condition by maintaining optimum levels of good bacteria. *PB 8®* contains eight strains of friendly bacteria per capsule, 14 billion count at the time of manufacture, and requires no refrigeration. NUTRITION NOW®, INC., 6350 NE Campus Dr., Vancouver, WA 98661-6877 (800) 929-0418   www.nutritionnow.com

SEX & NATURAL HORMONE THERAPY.

Symbiotropin™ (a Growth Hormone Releaser) was shown clinically to increase sexual potency/frequency by 32% and duration of penile erection by 44% within 90 days. *Testron SX*™ contains a variety of natural compounds to help support testosterone production. Safe and effective, it may be used by men and women for increased virility. For more information contact: NUTRACEUTICS CORP., 3317 NW Tenth Terrace, Suite 404, Fort Lauderdale, FL 33309 (800) 391-0114 (eastern U.S.) (800) 852-8582 (western U.S.)

AROMATHERAPY FACIAL CELL REJUVENATION. Rejuvenation Face Gel consists of a pure essential oil formula created specifically for cell rejuvenation and mature skin. It is excellent when used with our Rose-Lavender mist to balance and nurture the skin. For the body, choose *House Blend # 1,2,4, or 7* for cell and tissue health. The pure smells soothe the emotions which are reflected in the tissue. OIL LADY AROMATHERAPY®, 764 12th Avenue South, Naples, FL 34102 (941) 263-3451   FAX (941) 263-0898

FLAX SEED IN EASY TO USE FORM: Flax seed contains an abundant balance of Omega-3 and Omega-6 essential fatty acids, along with soluble and insoluble fiber and lignins. Therefore, it provides you with the best natural health package to balance, normalize and rejuvenate your body. Omega Life's *Fortified Flax* provides you with an easy to use flax meal with vitamins and minerals to help your body metabolize its wealth of benefits. It is also stabilized by a patented process to maintain freshness. *Fortified Flax* can be sprinkled on cereal, mixed with foods, bakery items, etc. and even added to your pet's food. You can also add to juice, their *Power Pack Energy Drink Mix*, which includes *Fortified Flax*, oat bran, barley, beta-carotene and lecithin or munch on *Omega Bars* to get your source of Omega-3's. OMEGA-LIFE, INC., PO Box 208, Brookfield, WI 53008-0208 (800) EAT-FLAX (328-3529).

MAIL ORDER CATALOG. Omega Nutrition's mail order catalogue carries many of the items recommended in "The Secrets of Staying Young," fresh from the farm and organic. Flax seeds, Essential Fatty Acid supplements including flax oil, Saw Palmetto Plus (with Pygeum,) Zinc, Vitamin E, hGH secretagogues, Royal Jelly, Gingko, Ginseng, Chromium, Natural Progesterone creams, Electrolytes, Enzymes and more. One stop shopping with reasonable prices. To receive a free catalog call OMEGA NUTRITION (800) 661-FLAX (661-3529).

BIOAVAILABLE PLANT ENZYMES:. TYME ZYME™ is a unique, highly concentrated enzyme formula for human consumption. *TYME ZYME*™ contains lipase, amylase, protease, cellulase and lactase enzymes in capsule form. *PROZYME*™ contains the protease, amylase, lipase and cellulase enzymes in powder form. Scientifically proven to increase the bioavailability and absorption of the vitamins, minerals, fatty acids and other vital nutrients in foods adding enzymes to your diet helps to slow the aging process. *PROZYME* is great to add to your cat or dog's diet too. PROZYME™ PRODUCTS, LTD. 6600 N. Lincoln Ave., Suite 312, Lincolnwood, IL 60645, (800)522-5537

WHEAT OR BARLEY GRASS SUPPLEMENTS: *Pines Wheat and Barley Grass* are grown a full 200 days in the rich Kansas soil and winter sunshine. This allows for optimum development of chlorophyll, long known for its ability to purify the blood and renew tissues. When harvested, these grasses are a naturally concentrated whole food, containing generous amounts of vitamins, minerals, anti-oxidants, protein and chlorophyll. The nutritional analysis of *Pines Wheat or Barley Grass* is much like that of a dark green leafy vegetable, but much more concentrated. Seven tablets or one teaspoon of powder, equals the nutrition found in a large serving of vegetables, such as a large spinach salad. Pines powders are 100% pure. the tablets are 98% pure and free of fillers or other ingredients that dilute the natural potency of the product. Pines has recently produced "Mighty Greens" which contains a blend of wheat, barley, rye and oat grass along with spirulina, alfalfa and other herbs. PINES INTERNATIONAL, INC., PO Box 1107, Lawrence, KS 66044 (800) 697-4637   www.Wheatgrass.com

YOUTH GIVING RHODODENDRON CAUCASICUM HERB. The herb consumed daily by one of the healthiest and longest living societies on earth - the people of the former Soviet Republic of Georgia. *Caucasicum*™ contains the Rhodogen™ root of a rare plant grown at 7000 feet above sea level. This supplement also contains grain kefir containing 11 probiotics as well as the complex of minerals extracted from the Glacial Milk waters of the Caucacus Mountains. Thirty years of research indicate that the Rhododendron improves physical abilities, increase activity of the cardiovascular system, and increase blood supply to the muscles and especially to the brain, increases resistance of the brain to imbalances due to chemical, physical and biological reasons. It also is an anti-bacterial while allowing the good probiotics to thrive. It acts as a detoxicant, is highly P-Vitamin active protecting against capillary fragility and is an excellent free-radical scavenger. QUEST IV HEALTH/ NUTRI-PET RESEARCH, 8 West Main St., Farmingdale, NJ 07727 (800) 360-3300

NEUROTRANSMITTER SUPPORT. *Restores*™ for adults and children contain the specific nutrients the brain must have to *replenish* low levels of vital neurotransmitters, a key element in reducing stress and improving brain function.. Made up of a special synergistic natural formulation of amino acids, vitamins and minerals, *Restores* also promotes increased serotonin, dopamine and endorphin levels. *Z-1* contains nutrients which support the body's natural cleansing actions and prevent unnecessary buildup of foods in the gastrointestinal tract during periods when metabolic rate is slow. *Z-1*™ is an excellent product for detoxification and for weight loss. It contains a proprietary ten stage oceanic phytoplankton complex, L-Carnitine and Rhodiola Rosea root extract which has also been shown to support the neurotransmitters and reduce symptoms of Parkinson disease and other aging illnesses. QUEST IV HEALTH/JOHN BOLUS, 2010 Alamanda Dr. #103, Naples, FL 34102 (941) 649-4964

SPROUTED SOY SUPPLEMENT AND PROGESTERONE CREAM. *REGENEZYME* powder (or caplets) is an all natural 100% organic, sprouted whole food concentrate. Sprouted soy does not contain the same allotype of provocative allergens common to soybean products. It is an excellent source of isoflavones and is beneficial to prostate health, menopausal symptoms and protein deficient diets. *ENDOCREME* serum or cream is a transdermal (percutaneous) delivery of natural progesterone and hormone precursors. These beneficial substances are more bioavailable to the body than in an orally used form.—especially due to *Endocreme's* proprietary delivery system ("Invisible Patch"). The products contain whole plant extracts, to provide a more synergistic and balancing effect. SEDNA SPECIALTY HEALTH PRODUCTS, P.O. Box 1453, Andrews, NC 28901 (800) 223-0858

ALL NATURAL BROAD-SPECTRUM MICRONUTRIENTS: The stresses of increasing micronutrient deficiencies in the diet can accelerate aging and depress the immune system. Ocean plants (seaweeds and kelp) naturally concentrate nature's richest source of chelated minor trace minerals and other micronutrients. Micronutrient supplementation has been shown to benefit allergies, immune response, hair growth, energy levels, and other symptoms of aging. *MICRO-MAX* is produced by the company that has innovated unique processing and blending techniques to preserve maximum micronutrient activity. SOURCE INCORPORTED, 101 Fowler Rd., N. Branford, CT 06471 (800) 232-2365   www.4source.com

SOLAR DISTILLATION ANTI-AGING ELIXIR. *SumerSun6 Renaissance*™ was developed by a nuclear physicist with over 200 national and international patents. It is composed of ATP and GTP in crystalline form that is capable of absorbing free energy. It is credited in its ability to increase energy while improving sleep. Renaissance is undergoing clinical studies to make the label statement claim: maintains healthy cholesterol levels and reduction of platelet aggregation. Renaissance contains chlorophyll as well as proteins and nucleotides from plant origin. It is 100% natural and is free of preservatives and artificial flavors, colors, etc. *Sumer gold* was discovered from ancient Sumerian tablets which describe an anti-aging elixir. *Sumer Gold* shares the same solar distillation process of Renaissance with a few refinements along the way. Its ability to address aging and genetic mutations takes place at the cellular level. Both products are taken sublingually and are 100% guaranteed. SUMER DISTRIBUTING, INC., 10801 Hammerly, Suite 150, Houston, TX 77043 (800) 324-5361

www.sumer.com

CERTIFIED ORGANIC WHEAT GRASS JUICE IN POWDER FORM. Convenient certified organic and Kosher wheat grass juice in freeze dried powder for increased stamina and physical performance. *Sweet Wheat*® is pure green energy direct from nature. High in zinc and vitamin A, vital to a healthy prostate gland for men and necessary to promote a healthy hormonal balance in women. It contains live enzymes for better digestion. *Sweet Wheat* also helps skin and eyesight as well as fortifying the immune system. This formula enhanced with crystalloid electrolytes is available as *Electra Green*. SWEET WHEAT, P.O. Box 187, Clearwater FL 33757-0187 (888) 227-9338   www.SweetWheat.com

FIGHT AGING WITH THE GREATEST FOODS ON EARTH. *Green Vibrance*™ is the superior restorative superfood containing hundreds of nutrients including organic cereal grass powders, sea vegetables, Hydrilla (a new fresh water green food), bee pollen, royal jelly, flax, green tea catechins extract and antioxidants. *Life Preserver*™ is a comprehensive total body antioxidant. *Joint Vibrance*™ is a safe and healthful treatment for arthritis containing Arthred™ hydrolyzed collagen, glucosamine, chondroitin and anti-inflammatory herbal extracts and special minerals to support enzymatic activity and tissue strength *Glycemic Vibrance*™ is a highly effective blood glucose stabilization formula suitable for all, especially persons with either elevated or depressed blood sugar. *Oryza Oil Tocotrienols* is a truly complete and hypoallergenic vitamin E complex. *Cholestatin* III™ wafers are a concentrate of plant sterols from soy beans known to block the absorption of cholesterol (and only cholesterol) from the gastrointestinal tract. Each wafer can block up to 300 mg. of cholesterol. TAAG, VIBRANT HEALTH, 432 Lime Rock Rd., Lakeville, CT 06039 (800) 242-1835

ALL NATURAL hGH PRECURSOR *Unitropin*™ contains natural substances that have been shown in clinical studies to cause the pituitary gland to secrete human growth hormone (hGH). *Unitropin*™ is based on research revealed by Dr. Ronald Klatz, M.D., who states that amino acids and some B vitamins cause the pituitary to release hGH. *Unitropin*™ combines the scientifically proven benefits of hGH research, B vitamins, (including Niacin, B6 and B12), amino acids (including choline, L-Arginine, L-Ornithine, L-Tyrosine, DL-Methionine, Alpha Ketoglutarate and Melatonin) with co-enzyme Q-10 and crystalloid electrolytes. *Unitropin*™ also contains a powerful, unique life-enhancing blend of herbs and extracts is an excellent anti-aging formula for both men and women. Herbs for sexual enhancement include *Tribulus terrestris* (to increase libido, recovery time from sexual activity, strength of erections and increase self-confidence in both men and women); *Muira puama* (a powerful aphrodisiac, nerve stimulant and overall mood enhancer); and *Korean Ginseng and Ashwaganda* (that reduce stress and bring the body into a state of equilibrium.) These ingredients create a powerful "global" formula that effects both body and mind creating a synergistic sense of well being. UNIVERSAL NETWORK, INCORPORATED, 5647 Beneva Road, Sarasota, FL 34332 (800) 446-0302

www. unitropin.com

SUPPORT HEALTHY PROSTATE FUNCTION. *PROSTA*LOGIC*™ is one of the most important nutritional supplements necessary for the prevention of prostate problems. *NEURO*LOGIC*™ is a brain enhancement formula developed by a leading neurologist, Dr. David Perlmutter. Taken daily, may be the perfect solution for the prevention of Alzheimer's disease. Also available, a unique, fast-acting, revolutionary arthritis (and other types of pain) relief cream called *GLUCOSAMATE*™ . WAKUNAGA OF AMERICA, 23501 Madero, Mission Viejo, CA 92691 (800) 825-7888

FORMULAS FOR MENTAL SUPPORT, ENERGY ENHANCEMEMT AND BODY STRUCTURE. For Mental Support: Ginkgo Biloba has been recommended for enhancing alertness, blood circulation and oxygen supply to the brain. *Super Ginkgo Biloba*™ blends 24% standardized Ginkgo Biloba extract with the antioxidant Pycnogenol® (a registered trademark of Horphag Research Ltd.) plus other natural nutrients known to support mental function and circulation throughout the body. Male Energy Enhancement: For thousands of years, Yohimbe Bark has been used to strengthen a man's energy level and enhance sexual drive. It was the first FDA approved herbal medicine for treating male impotence. Yohimbe's primary action is to increase blood flow to erectile tissue. *Super Yohimbe 1500*™ is an advanced formula containing Yohimbe Bark and fortified with essential male supportive herbs. Body Structure: *Super Glocosamine Complex 500* mg features Chondroitin Sulfate and MSM (Methylsulfonylmethane), nutrients recognized for their roles in promoting healthy maintenance of the body's physical structure including muscles, joints and connective tissue. USA NUTRITIONALS INC, 280 Adams Blvd., Farmingdale, NY 11735 (800) 722-7570   www.USANutritionals.com

AGED GARLIC EXTRACT, GREENS AND ACIDOPHILUS: Choosing an appropriate garlic supplement can be a confusing process. Actually, there are 4 choices: (1) heat distilled garlic oil in softgels, (2)heat dehydrated garlic seasoning powder in capsules/tablets, (3) garlic oil macerates and (4) *KYOLIC odorless Aged Garlic Extract*™. All garlic supplements probably have some nutritional value, but oils and powders do not contain significant amounts of water soluble compounds which are essential to retain all of the benefits of garlic. Garlic oils and powders contain smelly oil soluble sulphur compounds which cause pungent garlic odor as well as harsh oxidizing side effects.. Since the development of *Kyolic*® almost four decades ago, more research has been done on this Aged Garlic Extract, than on all other garlic supplements combined. *Kyolic*® is also covered by more than a dozen patents and patents pending worldwide. See the chapter "Garlic" for the benefits of Aged Garlic Extract (AGE). The makers of *Kyolic*® also provide a comprehensive powdered "green" drink which includes young barley and wheat grasses grown in the pristine Nasu Highlands in Japan, cooked brown rice, chlorella from natural mineral springs, and kelp from the Northern Pacific. This combination provides you with a daily balanced amount of greens. Also necessary for the body, is the addition of L.acidophilus, B.bifidum and B.longum strains of live "friendly" bacteria found in *Kyo-Dophilus*® used in 30,000 hospitals and clinics. This product is heat stable (needs no refrigeration) and therefore is excellent for traveling. It is human grade therefore is bioavailable in the digestive tract. This makes it an safe product for all ages.. Another product, *Acidophilase*™ combines the "friendly" bacteria with enzymes, amylase, lipase and protease. These products are all yeast, sodium and dairy free and are available at your local stores or through WAKUNAGA OF AMERICA, 23501 Madero, Mission Viejo, CA 92691 (800) 825-7888

The statements in this chapter of paragraph descriptions may not have been evaluated by the Food and Drug Administration (FDA) to treat, diagnose, cure or prevent any disease. The health claims are provided for informational purposes only.

BIBLIOGRAPHY

-Abe, S. and Kaneda, T., *The effect of edible seaweeds on cholesterol metabolism in rats. In Proceedings of the Seventh International Seaweed Symposium*, Wiley and Sons, NY, pp. 562-565, 1972

-Aihara, Herman, *Acid & Akaline*, George Oshawa Microbiotic Foundation, 1986

-Albuirmeileh, N. et al., *Suppression of Cholesterogenesis by Kyolic and S.-Ally Cysteine*, The FASEB Jnl, 5:A1756, 1991

-Anderson, Dr. Richard, ND, NMD, *Cleanse & Purify Thyself*, R. Anderson, 1988

-Aso H., *Induction of interferon and activation of NK cells and macrophages in mice by oral administration of Ge-132, an organic germanium compound*, Microbiol Immunol, 1985, 8(5); 352-353

-Bach, Nelson, USA, *Finding Balance Through Flower Remedies*, Healthy & Natural, Vol. 2, No. 1

-Balch, James, M.D., *Prescriptions for Nutritional Healing*, Avery Publishing, 1996

-Berg, W., Bother, C., and Schneider, H.J.: *Experimental and Clinical Studies Concerning the Influence of Natural Substances on the Crystallization of Calcium Oxalate*, Urologe 21:52-58, 1982

-Blaylock, Russel L. M.D.., *Excitotoxins, The Taste That Kills*, Health Press, 1997

-Breuninger, Heather, *Are Enzymes The Key to Boosting Immunity?*, Natural Foods Merchandiser, June 1993

-Bricklin, Mark, *Natural Healing*, Rodale Press, 1976

-Caporase N., Smith S.M. and Eng R.H.K., *Antifungal Activity in Human Urine and Serum After Ingestion of Garlic (Allium sativum)*, antimicrobial Agents and Chemotherapy, 23: 700-702, 1983

-Chapman, J.B., MD and Perry, Edward L., MD, *The Biochemic Handbook*, Formur, Inc., 1976

-Choi, Steve S., *Royal Jelly, the Fountain of Youth*, Health World, Sept/Oct, 1991

-Cichoke, Anthony J., MA, DC, DACBN, *Aged Garlic Extract*, Health & Natural, Vol 2, No.1, 1995

-Cichoke, Anthony J., MA, DC, DACBN, *Healing Powers of Aged Garlic Extract*, Townsend Letter for Doctors, June 1994

-Cichoke, Dr. A.J., *Enzymes*, Lets Live, June 1994

-Cichoke, A.J., DC., *Systemic Enzyme Therapy*, The American Chiropractor,April, 1991

-Cichoke, Anthony J., *Bee Pollen, The Latest Buzz on the Power of Nectar*, Body, Mind, Spirit, Feb. - March, 1995

-Cichoke, A.J., DC, *Fight Back Pain with Enzymes*, Lets Live, May 1994

-Clark, Linda, M.A., *Enzymes can help your health*, Lets Live, June 1977

-Cutler, Richard, G., PhD, *Antioxidants and Aging*, American Journal of Clinical Nutrition, 1991

-Cowley, Goeffrey, *Cancer & Diet*, Newsweek: 60-66, November 30, 1998

-*Daily Vitamin D Can Reduce Fracture Risk*, Medical Tribune, Aug. 20, 1992

-De Vries, Jan, *Traditional Home & Herbal Remedies*, Mainstream Publishing, 1989

-Dittmar, Mary Jane, *Getting The Inside Track on Enzymes*, Health Foods Business, Jan. 1987

-Erasmus, Udo, *The Value of Fresh Flax Oil*, Lipid Letter, Issue No.3

-Fallon, Sally W and Enig, Mary G., *Soy Products for Dairy Products? Not So Fast.*, Health Freedom News, Sept, 1995

-Frank, Benjamin S.M.D., *Nucleic Acid and Anti-Oxidant Therapy of Aging and Degeneration*, Rainstone Publishing, 1977

-Gittleman, Ann Louise, *Super Nutrition for Menopause*, Pocket Books, 1993

-Goldberg, S.L., *The Use of Water Soluble Chlorophyll in Oral Sepsis*, Am. J. Surg 62:117-123, 1943

Goldberg, M.P.D., D.C., *Use of Live Enzyme Whole Food in a Chiropractic Practice: One Practicioner's Experience*, American Chiropracter, July 1990

-Golden T, and Burke, J.F., *Effective Management of Offensive Odors.*, Gastroenterology 31:260-265, 1956

-Gruskin, G., *Chlorophyll -Its Therapeutic Place in Acute and Suppurative Disease*, Am. J. Surg 49:49-54, 1940

-Heimlich, Jane, *What Your Doctor Won't Tell You*, Phillips Publishing, Apr. 1992

-Holly, Cory, DN, *Your Liver, Your Life*, Alive Magazine, #137

-Howell, Dr. Edward, *Enzyme Nutrition*, Avery Publishing, 1985

-Hughes, David B., Hoover, Dallas G., *Bifidobacteria: Their Potential for Use in American Dairy Products*, Food Technology, April 1991

-Huntoon, Jenefer Scripps, N.D., *Consumer Education Series: Enzymes*, Health Foods Business, March 1989

-I-San Lin, Dr. Robert, *Garlic & Health*, International Academy of Health and Fitness, Inc., 1994

-Imada O., *Toxicity Aspect of Garlic*, In abstract of the First World Congress on the Health Significance of Garlic and Garlic Constituents, p 47, 1990

-*In Health*, Naturopathic Physician, Vol 2, No.2

-Jarvis, DC, *Folk Medicine*, Fawcett Crest, 1958

-Jensen, Bernard, Ph.D., *Chlorella, Jewel of the Far East*, Bernard Jensen, 1992

-Jensen, Bernard, Ph.D., *Foods That Heal*, Avery Publishing, 1993

-Jesswith, Sophia, *Living food*, Alive magazine, #148
-Kamen, Betty, Ph.D., *Bee Pollen" From Principles to Practice*, Health Food Business, April 1991
-Kamen, Betty, Ph.D., *Avoiding and Reversing Osteoporosis*, Natural Solutions, Vol ii, Issue I, Winter, 1994
-Konishi F, Tanaka K, Himeno K et al, *Antitumor effect induced by a hot Water extract of Chlorella vulgaris (CE): resistance to Meth-A Tumor Growth Mediated by CE - induced Polymorphonuclear Leukocytes.*, Cancer Immunol Immunother 19:73-78, 1985
-Kotulak, Ronald, Gorner, Peter, *Aging on Hold*, Tribune Publishing, 1992
-Kulawiec, Matthew H., *Keep the Colon Clean*, Alive Magazine, #157 Nov. 1995
-Lau, B.H.S., Ong, P., Tosk, J.,*Macrohpage chemiluminescence modulated by Chinese medicinal herbs Astragalus membranaceus and Ligustrum lucidum*, Phytotherapy Res. 3:148-153, 1989
-Lau, Benjamin H.S., MD, PhD, *Garlic Research Update*, Odyssey Publishing, 1991
-Lau, Benjamin H.S.,MD., PhD., *Detoxifying, Radioprotective and Phagocyte-enhancing effects of Garlic*, International Clinical Nutrition Review, Jan, 1989, Vol 9 No. 1
-Lau, B.H.S., et al., *Superiority of Intralesional Immunotherapy with C-Cynebacterium parvum and Allium sativum in Control of Murine Transitional Cell Carcinoma*, The Journal. of Urology, 136:701-705, 1986
-Lawson,L.D. and Hughes, B.G., *Characterization of Formation of Allicin and Other Thiosulfinates from Garlic*, Planta Medica 58: 345-350, 1992
-Lee, Lita, *Prostate Problems*, Earthletter, Winter, 1993
-Lee, Lita, Menopause, *Osteoporosis & the ERT Fairy Tale*, Earthletter, Vol 4 No. 2, Summer 1994
-Lee, Lita, *Anti-tumor properties of natural progesterone*, Earthletter, Spring, 1993
-Lee, Lita, *Cyclic seizures due to estrogen toxicity*, Earthletter, Summer, 1993
-Lee, Lita, *Estrogen Mimics: Xenoestrogens* Earthletter, Fall, 1994
-Lee, Lita PhD, *Radiation Protection Manual*, Grassroots Network, 1990
-Lewin, Renate, *Rediscovering Flax: Essential Fats and Fiber in a Single Package*, Lets' Live, Jan. 1989
-Liu, J. et al., *Inhibition of 7,12-dimethylbenz(a)anthracene-induced Mammary Tumors and DNA Adducts by Garlic Powder*, Carcinogenesis, 13: 1847-1851, 1992
-Loomis, Howard, D.C. and Sutliff, Kris, PhD, Improve Digestion with Plant Enzymes, The American Chiropractor, Feb. 1990
-Loomis, Howard, D.C., *Practical Applications of Enzyme Nutrition: Improve Digestion with Plant Enzymes*, The American Chiropractor, Feb. 1990
-McAuliff, Jill, *Can Herbs the the answer to the problem of Hair Loss?*, Healthy and Natural, Vol. 2 No. 2
-Mann, John, Kelly, Aidan A., Ph.D., Dravnieks, Dzintar, Ph.D., *Secrets of Life Extension*, And/Or Press, 1978
-McClure, Steven, N.D., *Raw Power Plus*, Reflections, Spring, 1988
-Messina, Mark, PhD,Virginia Messina, RD,Setchell, Kenneth, D.R., PhD, *The Simple Soybean and Your Health*, Avery Publishing, 1994
-Mertlew, Gillian, N.D., *Electrolytes, The Spark of Life*, Nature's Publishing, 1994
-Meyerowitz, Steve, *Wheatgrass, Nature's Finest Medicine*, The Sprout House, Inc., 1991
-Mitsuoka, Tomotari PhD, *Intestinal Flora and Aging*, Nutrition Reviews, Vol 50 No. 12
-Morgenthaler, John, & Joy, Dan, *Better Sex through Chemistry*, Smart Publishing, 1993
-Murray, Frank, *Royal Jelly, It's not just for queen bees*, Better Nutrition, August, 1990
-Nakayama S., Yoshisa S., Horao Y, et al., *Cytoprotective activity of components of garlic, ginseng, and ciuwijia on hepatocyte injury induced by carbon tetrachloride in vitro*, Hiroshima J. Med Sci, 1985; 5:460-461
-Negeshi, T. Arimosto, S., Nashizaki, C. et al., *Inhibitory Effect of Chlorophyll on the Genotoxicity of 3-amino-1-methyl5H=pyridol (4,3-b)-indole (Try P-2)*, Carcinogenesis 10:145-149, 1989
-Nesaretnam, K., et. Al., *Tocotrienols inhibit the growth of human breast cancer cells irrespective of estrogen receptor status*, Lipids, 33(5): 461-469, May 1998
-Nishino H., Nishino A., Takayasu J. et al., *Antitumor-Promoting Activity of Allixin, a Stress Compound Produced by Garlic*, Cancer J. 3"20-21, 1990
-*Nutritional Enzymes: Questions and Answers*, National Enzyme Co., July 1993
-Ozer, N.K., et.al. *New roles of low density lipoproteins and vitamin E in the pathogenesis of atherosclerosis*, Biochem Mol. Biol. Int., 35(1): 117-24, January , 1995
-Peat, Ray, *The Progesterone Deception*, Townsend Letter for Doctors, Nov., 1987.
-Petkov, V.D., Yonkov, D., Mosharoff, A., et al., *Effects of Alcohol Aqueous Extract from Rhodiola rosea L. Roots on Learning and Memory.*, ACT Physiologica Et Pharmacologica Bulgarica, Vol. 12, No. 3, Sofia, 1986
-Pierson, Dr. Herbert, *Synopsis of Designer foods III Phytochemicals in Garlic, Soy & Licorice*, Georgetown University, June 2, 1994
-Qureshi, AA., et.al. *Response of hypercholesterolemic subjects to administration of tocotrienols.*, Lipids, 30(12): 1171-7, December, 1995
-Quillin, P., *Healing Nutrients*, Random House, 1987
-Quinn, Dick, *Left For Dead*, Quinn Publishing, 1994

-Qureshi, A.A. et al., *Inhibition of Cholesterol Synthesis by Kyolic (Aged Garlic Extract) and S-Allyl Cysteine in a Hypercholesterolemic Model*, Abstracts of the FirstWorld Congress on the Health Significance of Garlic and Garlic Constituents, pp17, 1990

-Ratcliff, J.D., *Enzymes, Medicine's Bright Hope*, The Reader's Digest, June 1961

-Rector-Page, Linda, ND, PhD, *Detoxification & Body Cleansing*, Healthy Healing Publications, 1993

-Rochefort, Henri, *Do Anti-Estrogens and Anti-progestins act as Hormone-antagonists or recepter targeted drugs in Breast Cancer?*, Trends in Pharmaceutical Sciences, April 1987

-Roderick, Dave, *Skin Therapy and Osteoporosis*, Clinical Nutrition News, 1995

-Rogers, Sherry, M.D., *Enzymes fight cancer*, Lets Live, May 1995

-Rothschild, P.R., Ordoniz, L., *Absorption Study with SOC/CAT®*, Univ. Labs Press

-St. Claire, Debra, *American and European Herbology*, Healthy & Natural, Vol. 2, #1.

-Sardi, Bill, *Healthy Vision*, NFM's Nutrition Science News, Oct. 1996

-Schecter, Steven R., *Welcome to the Pollen Nation*, Healthy & Natural Vol.2 Issue 3

-Schwontkowski, Dr. Donna, *Herbal Treasures of the Rainforest*, Healthy & Natural , Oct. 1994

-Sheer, James F. *Dethrone aging with Royal Jelly*, Better Nutrition, June, 1995

-Seibold, Ronald L., M.S., *Cereal Grass What's In It For You!*, Wilderness Community Education Foundation, Inc., 1990

-Sellman, Sherrill, *Hormone Heresy*, Get Well International, 1998

-SGP, *The Therapeutic Garlic*. Osaka, The Wakunaga Pharmaceutical Company, 1987

-SGP, *Wakunaga Probiotics For Maintaining a Healthy Intestinal Flora for Normal Digestive Function*, The Wakunaga Pharmaceutical Corp., 1995

-Spake, Amanda, *Maverick Scientist Devra Lee Davis is Afraid She Knows the Answer*, Health, October, 1995

-Spectrum Naturals, *Basic Facts on Fats and Oils*, Spectrum, 1993

-Strause, Linda, Saltman, Paul et al., *Spinal Bone Loss in Postmenopausal Women Supplemented with Calcium and Trace Minerals*. Journal. of Nutrition, 1994 p 1060-1064

-Sumiyoshi, H. and Wargovich, M.J., *Chemoprevention of 1,2-dimethylhydrazine-induced Colon Cancer in Mice by Naturally Occurring Organosulfur Compounds*, Cancer Research., 50:5084-5087, 1990

-Suzuki, F, Pollard RB, *Prevention of suppressed gamma-interferon production in thermally injured mice by administration of novel organogermanium compound Ge-132*, J. Interferon Research, 1984; 4:223-233

-Tadi, Padama P.M.S., Teel, Robert W., PhD., and Lau, Benjamin, H.S., MD, PhD, *Anticandidal and Anticarcinogenic Potentials of Garlic*, Integrated Therapies, 1990

-Takeyama, H. et al., *Growth Inhibition and Modulation of Cell Markers of Melanoma by S-allyCysteine*, Oncology, 50:63-39, 1993

-Tanaka K, Konishi F, Mimeno K et al., *Augmentation of antitumor resistance by a strain of unicellular green algae, Chlorella vulgaris.*, Cancer Immunol Immunother 17:90-94, 1984

-Teas J., *The consumption of seaweed as a protective factor in the etiology of breast cancer.*, Med. Hypotheses 7:601-613, 1981

-Teas, J., *The dietary intake of Laminaria, a brown seaweed and breast cancer prevention.*, Nutritional Cancer 4:217-222, 1983

-Teoh, M.K., et. al., *Protection by tocotrienols against hypercholesterolaemia and atheroma*, Med. J. Malaysia, 49(3): 244-62, September, 1994

-Terwel, L. and Van der Hoeven, J.C.M., *Antimutagenic Activity of Some Naturally Occurring Compounds Towards Cigarette-smoke Condensate and Benzoalpyrene in the Salmonella/microsome Assay.*, Mutation Res 152:1-4, 1985

-Tho, L.L. and Candlish, J.K., *Superoxide Dismutase and Glutathione Peroxidase Activities in Erythrocytes as Indices of Oxygen Loading Disease: A Survey of 100 cases.*, Biochemical Medicine and Metabolic Biology, 38, 365-373, 1987

-Thomas, John, *Young Again! How to Reverse the Aging Process*, Plexus Press, 1994

-Thomas, Richard, *The Essiac Report*, Alternative Treatment Information Network, 1993

-Tobe, John, *Enzymes: Nature's Metabolizers*, Cancer Forum, Summer 1995

-Tosk, J., Lau, B.H.S., Jui, Pl, Myers, R.C. and Torrey, R.R., *Chemiluminescence in a macrophage cell line modulated by biological response modifiers.*, J.Leukocyte Biol. 46:103-108, 1989

-Vogel, A. MD, *Book of Fourteen Amazing Herbal Medicines*, Keats Publishing, 1990

-Yamagishi, Yoshio, Yaguchi, Isamu, Kenmoku, Yukie, *Clinical Studies on Chlorella*, "Nippon Iji Shimpo", 17-18 (No. 2196), May 28, 1966

-Yu t-H and Wuc-m, *Stability of Allicin in Garlic Juice.*, J. Food Sci. 54: 977-981, 1989

-Yeh, Y.Y., et al., *Hypolipidemic Effects of Garlic Extract in Vivo and in Vitro*, Absteracts of the First World Congress on the Health Significance of Garlic and Garlic Constituents, pp.37, 1990

-Ziegler, Jan, *Just the Flax, Ma'am: Researchers Testing Linseed*, Journal of the National Cancer Inst. 86(23):1746-1748, Dec. 7, 1994

172

INDEX

A-B

acid/alkaline, 24, 46, 162
Acidophilus, 30, 31, 164, 183
acne, 71, 95, 97, 98, 100
adrenal, 93, 97, 99, 100, 117, 136
adrenals, 24, 93, 136, 143
AFB, 110
AGE, 103, 147, 169
age spots, 4, 51, 103, 104
Aged Garlic Extract, 26, 81, 82, 83, 84, 115, 169, 170, 172
AIDS, 81
Albert Schweitzer, 81
alcohol, 25, 27, 30, 72, 74, 114, 117, 120, 126, 128, 130, 132, 133, 135, 159
alfalfa, 26, 118, 159, 166
algae, 65, 66, 67, 68, 90, 92, 112, 172
alkaline, 24, 25, 26, 27, 37, 38, 39, 46, 162
alkalize, 26, 64
allergies, 19, 47, 48, 51, 65, 78, 89, 143, 145, 167
allicin, 83
allopathic, 29
almonds, 4, 71
aloe, 4, 26, 71, 91, 108, 138, 159
aluminum, 36, 41, 126, 130
Alzheimer's, 41, 168
amino acids, 17, 19, 32, 41, 42, 46, 65, 67, 69, 72, 82, 91, 96, 111, 112, 113, 120, 127, 128, 129, 133, 136, 160, 162, 166, 168
ANDRO, 98, 99
anemia, 28, 41, 42
antibiotics, 30, 72
antibodies, 65
antifungal, 59, 81
antioxidants, 3, 17, 19, 45, 61, 64, 69, 71, 73, 168
anxiety, 99, 118, 119, 120, 126, 136, 137, 160
aosain, 90
aphrodisiac, 133
arteries, 42, 52, 57, 86, 115, 116, 160, 163
arteriosclerosis, 115
artery, 42, 57, 115
arthritis, 3, 5, 38, 52, 59, 64, 80, 87, 104, 105, 106, 107, 114, 144, 160, 168
aspartame, 128
Aspergillus, 110
asthma, 52, 59, 65, 72, 73, 79
athlete, 41, 42, 53, 80, 92
ATP, 3, 69, 84, 103, 167
back pain, 105, 130, 163
bacteria, 19, 23, 25, 27, 30, 31, 32, 33, 36, 48, 59, 62, 64, 72, 87, 89, 106, 131, 164, 169, 183
baldness, 60, 66, 107
barley, 15, 62, 63, 64, 65, 68, 90, 110, 116, 123, 165, 166, 169
Bee pollen, 132
bees, 72, 105, 171
bentonite, 28
Bifidobacterium, 30

bioavailable, 48, 169
bioflavonoids, 4, 63, 73, 112, 125, 138, 163
Black Cohosh, 96
blindness, 28, 113
blood, 3, 17, 19, 20, 21, 23, 24, 26, 27, 29, 41, 42, 43, 47, 49, 52, 53, 56, 57, 58, 59, 61, 62, 63, 64, 66, 68, 75, 77, 78, 81, 82, 84, 85, 86, 87, 93, 95, 100, 103, 104, 105, 106, 107, 108, 109, 111, 114, 115, 116, 117, 118, 120, 121, 123, 124, 126, 127, 129, 132, 134, 141, 142, 159, 161, 162, 163, 166, 168, 169
blood clots, 52, 108, 118
blood thinner, 108, 118
bone, 24, 58, 72, 74, 95, 98, 100, 104, 106, 122, 123, 124, 125, 147, 149, 160
Borage, 104
boron, 163
bowel, 19, 27, 59
brain, 9, 17, 20, 24, 41, 43, 50, 72, 74, 76, 79, 85, 106, 108, 109, 113, 119, 120, 121, 127, 128, 129, 133, 136, 141, 159, 163, 166, 168, 169
breast, 60, 62, 66, 71, 94, 97, 98, 100, 109, 110, 117, 171, 172
brittle nails, 59, 90

C-D

caffeine, 25, 27, 89, 91, 126, 130, 132, 133
Calc. Fluor, 105, 138
calcium, 24, 35, 37, 41, 42, 48, 49, 62, 64, 66, 68, 71, 82, 96, 105, 122, 123, 124, 125, 130, 163
cancer, 27, 31, 49, 50, 52, 55, 57, 58, 60, 62, 63, 66, 68, 72, 73, 77, 79, 80, 82, 83, 86, 90, 93, 94, 109, 110, 111, 116, 117, 127, 131, 142, 171, 172
Candida, 36, 48, 84
capillaries, 41, 72, 103, 107
capsicum, 26
carbohydrates, 17, 18, 26, 32, 46, 69, 96, 106, 162
carcinogen, 110
Cascara Sagrada, 29
catalase, 50, 84
cataracts, 5, 111, 112
caucasicum, 3, 11, 85, 106, 114
cell, 17, 22, 24, 33, 37, 40, 48, 50, 51, 55, 57, 61, 66, 67, 68, 72, 73, 75, 78, 81, 89, 90, 91, 93, 108, 110, 111, 120, 127, 138, 161, 163, 164, 165, 172
cellulase, 46, 165
cellulite, 4, 75, 92
cereal grass, 25, 27, 61, 62, 63, 64, 65, 69, 136
chelate, 112, 121
chemical sensitivity, 26
Chlorella, 15, 27, 62, 63, 65, 66, 67, 68, 70, 170, 171, 172
chlorophyll, 15, 26, 56, 62, 63, 64, 66, 68, 69, 166, 167
cholesterol, 3, 19, 26, 52, 56, 59, 62, 66, 68, 71, 73, 74, 76, 77, 80, 84, 86, 87, 95, 98, 99, 115,

116, 117, 121, 131, 132, 134, 162, 163, 167, 168, 170
Chondroitin sulfate, 106, 162
chromium, 36, 42
circulation, 20, 41, 62, 79, 84, 86, 109, 118, 121, 162, 169
clot, 58, 108
coffee, 25, 117, 161
colitis, 27
collagen, 50, 89, 90, 106, 107, 116, 160, 162, 168
colloidal, 33, 40
constipation, 25, 26, 27, 80, 94, 131, 138
copper, 36, 37, 41, 56, 82, 124, 159
corn, 21, 55, 56, 110
cross linking, 51
Crystalloid, 40, 43, 91
cysts, 94
dairy, 25, 27, 31, 38, 48, 64, 121, 123, 137, 169
Damiana, 109, 132, 133, 134
degenerative disease, 5, 9, 23, 24, 45, 57, 61
dehydration, 90
depression, 3, 26, 59, 86, 87, 94, 95, 97, 100, 118, 119, 120, 123, 129, 133, 135, 137, 143, 160, 161
detoxify, 24, 45, 51, 161
DHEA, 98, 99, 100
DHT, 130, 132
diabetes, 52, 57, 60, 147
diarrhea, 25, 29, 79, 81
Dick Quinn, 108, 138
digestion, 4, 17, 18, 20, 21, 26, 31, 45, 46, 47, 48, 49, 52, 53, 75, 89, 125, 164, 167
digestive enzymes, 31, 45, 46, 48, 49, 53, 72
digestive tract, 23, 27, 28, 53, 59, 169
Dimitry M. Rossiyski, M.D, 86
diverticulitis, 27
dizziness, 26, 121
DNA, 57, 67, 72, 110
Dong Quai, 97
dopamine, 121, 126, 129, 166
Dr. Benjamin Lau, 62
Dr. Edward Howell, 45
Dr. Linda Rector Page, 98
Dr. Manfred Steins, 115
Dr. Sherry Rogers, 52
Dr. Tariq Abdullah, 81
Dr. Walter Willet, 56
Dr. Wm. Lowe Mundy, 145
dry skin, 59, 90, 91

E-F

ears, 59, 121
Echinacea, 26, 132, 134
EFAs, 58, 59, 60, 116
ejaculation, 130, 134
elastase, 89, 90
elastin, 89, 90
elderly, 52, 63, 140
electrolytes, 13, 22, 25, 32, 33, 36, 40, 42, 50, 91, 116, 124, 163, 164, 167, 168

elimination, 17, 20, 26, 28, 29, 86, 89, 114
emotional problems, 121, 143
endocrine, 74, 95, 96, 98
enzyme, 26, 33, 40, 41, 45, 46, 47, 48, 49, 50, 51, 52, 53, 62, 66, 82, 86, 89, 90, 96, 99, 106, 110, 125, 130, 161, 165, 168
enzyme inhibitors, 49
epidermis, 90
Epsom salts, 29
erectile, 109
erection, 42, 134, 165
ERT, 94, 171
essential fatty acids, 13, 46, 55, 58, 98, 103, 116, 121, 130, 133, 136, 137, 161, 165
estrogen, 4, 24, 60, 75, 90, 93, 94, 96, 97, 98, 109, 117, 122, 123, 124, 125, 171
excitotoxins, 126, 128, 129
exercise, 20, 53, 60, 84, 120, 130, 138, 147, 148, 149, 150, 151, 152, 155
eyes, 20, 30, 53, 106, 112
fast, 21, 25, 98, 135, 148, 168
fatigue, 19, 26, 41, 94, 106, 113, 118, 120, 123, 130, 135, 136, 163, 164, 183
fatty acids, 13, 14, 19, 46, 55, 56, 58, 59, 60, 69, 98, 103, 107, 116, 118, 121, 130, 133, 136, 137, 161, 165
Fennel, 29
fermented soy, 49
fiber, 19, 20, 21, 46, 59, 71, 89, 130, 131, 132, 137, 165
flax, 52, 56, 59, 96, 116, 118, 129, 161, 165, 168
flower, 27, 76, 80, 103, 112, 119, 121, 135, 136, 137
food allergies, 47, 89
free radical scavengers, 39
free radicals, 43, 50, 61, 64, 70, 71, 73, 84, 87, 104

G-K

garlic, 26, 27, 55, 80, 81, 82, 83, 84, 105, 108, 109, 115, 126, 132, 136, 138, 169, 171
gastrointestinal, 46, 66, 166, 168
genetic, 3, 21, 60, 69, 70, 89, 107, 167
germanium, 82, 170
ginkgo, 79, 99, 115, 119, 121
ginseng, 21, 96, 97, 99, 100, 118, 119, 121, 132, 133, 134, 136, 171
GLA, 60, 104, 118
Glaucoma, 113
glucosamine, 106, 107, 168
glucose, 19, 69, 75, 111, 161, 168
gout, 3, 4, 86, 87, 114, 115
grain, 19, 20, 31, 48, 64, 85, 166
Grape Seed, 87
gray hair, 66, 74
green papaya, 51
green tea, 110, 168
growth depressant, 49
hair loss, 59, 60, 100, 107
headaches, 26, 28, 29, 94, 97, 99, 100, 113, 121, 128

healing crisis, 53

heart, 3, 8, 9, 20, 42, 50, 52, 55, 56, 57, 58, 59, 60, 77, 79, 80, 86, 87, 94, 98, 108, 115, 116, 123, 139, 147, 162

heart palpitations, 123

heavy metal, 25, 80, 83, 121, 126, 129, 163

herbs, 26, 27, 29, 79, 80, 91, 97, 101, 103, 116, 118, 119, 121, 127, 133, 134, 136, 137, 158, 161, 163, 164, 166, 168, 169, 171, 183

HGH, 4, 74, 75, 78

homeopathic, 4, 30, 31, 40, 76, 80, 101, 103, 105, 118, 132, 159, 160, 164

homeostasis, 36, 39, 40, 124, 163

honey, 38, 70, 73, 85, 104

hormones, 24, 26, 60, 65, 72, 75, 93, 95, 98, 115, 120, 124, 127, 130, 133, 162

hot flashes, 4, 93, 97, 117, 118

Hunza's, 35

hydrochloric acid, 45, 52

hydrogenated, 56, 57, 107

immune system, 13, 15, 19, 23, 27, 29, 30, 36, 39, 47, 50, 59, 62, 66, 67, 71, 72, 73, 74, 78, 81, 82, 84, 92, 104, 107, 111, 119, 131, 135, 136, 141, 143, 144, 145, 160, 161, 167

impotence, 96, 97, 108, 130, 132

inflammation, 79, 104, 106, 132, 134, 160

influenza, 30, 84

insomnia, 72, 94, 99, 100, 118, 119, 130

intestinal flora, 30

intestine, 18, 19, 30, 31, 46, 47

iodine, 36, 66, 96

iron, 37, 41, 42, 49, 62, 63, 82, 96, 124

irritability, 99, 100, 124, 132

James Balch, M.D., 121

James Jamieson, 78, 96

joints, 38, 40, 42, 104, 105, 114, 169

jojoba, 74

kale, 112, 123

kelp, 15, 66, 68, 92, 105, 136, 167, 169

kidney, 25, 29, 57, 64, 72, 114, 161

kidney stones, 64

Kyolic, 81, 83, 115, 169

L-R

L.O. Pilgeram, 52

LDL, 20, 57, 71, 115, 116

leaky gut, 30, 47, 57

lecithin, 26, 56, 72, 76, 120, 163, 165

lethargy, 135

leuteinizing hormone, 134

libido, 98, 99, 130, 132, 133, 134, 164, 168

licorice, 26, 27, 97, 118, 136

ligaments, 42, 149, 159

lignin, 59

linoleic, 59, 60

linolenic, 59, 118

lipase, 46, 50, 52, 165, 169

liver, 20, 26, 27, 29, 52, 53, 57, 60, 61, 72, 74, 76, 77, 83, 84, 89, 90, 94, 98, 100, 103, 110, 114, 116, 118, 143, 161

Lobelia, 29

lungs, 20, 147

lycopene, 110

lymph, 26, 29, 104, 130

lymph glands, 26

lymphatic, 47

Maca, 96

macrophages, 31, 62, 71, 170

Macular degeneration, 112, 113

magnesium, 37, 41, 42, 49, 62, 66, 71, 82, 92, 96, 105, 111, 123, 124, 125, 137, 163

maldigestion, 20

male hormone, 97

malnutrition, 27

manganese, 37, 42, 124

margarine, 9, 56, 107

meat, 25, 39, 41, 48, 49, 64, 69, 130, 132, 137

melatonin, 24, 75, 100, 118, 168

membranes, 17, 29, 31, 82, 89, 120, 131

memory, 20, 41, 74, 76, 79, 120, 121, 161, 163

menopausal, 89, 93, 95, 96, 117, 118, 124, 147, 163, 167

menopause, 93, 96, 97, 117, 123, 124, 126, 149, 164, 183

mercury, 51, 83

metabolic enzymes, 46, 48, 53

metabolism, 21, 24, 30, 39, 42, 52, 55, 57, 58, 62, 66, 98, 110, 124, 125, 161, 170

Methionine Reductase, 50, 51

micronutrient, 65, 66, 167

migraines, 59

minerals, 13, 17, 18, 19, 22, 25, 26, 32, 35, 36, 37, 38, 39, 40, 41, 42, 43, 45, 46, 49, 50, 56, 58, 61, 62, 66, 69, 72, 82, 85, 91, 92, 96, 104, 107, 112, 119, 123, 124, 125, 133, 136, 137, 149, 157, 158, 159, 160, 162, 163, 165, 166, 167, 168

muscle, 4, 28, 42, 50, 60, 69, 74, 75, 98, 109, 116, 147, 149, 150, 155, 160, 163

mutation, 64

myofibrosis, 38

NaPCA, 91

natural progesterone, 94, 95, 117, 164, 167, 171, 183

naturopathic, 29, 118

nausea, 26, 101

neurotransmitters, 65, 119, 120, 127, 129, 136, 166

nose, 133

nuclear, 70, 167

nutrients, 8, 17, 18, 20, 21, 23, 30, 36, 42, 46, 48, 49, 56, 57, 58, 61, 62, 64, 66, 68, 69, 72, 74, 79, 82, 91, 92, 95, 96, 111, 125, 135, 157, 158, 161, 162, 163, 164, 165, 166, 168, 169

nutritional yeast, 32, 76, 105

olive oil, 26, 29, 58, 71

organs, 20, 23, 24, 25, 26, 38, 53, 57, 67, 70, 74, 97, 104, 132, 141, 143, 161

osteoblasts, 122, 125

osteoclasts, 122, 125

osteoporosis, 4, 95, 98, 122, 123, 125, 134, 147, 163
ovaries, 93
oxygen, 17, 20, 26, 39, 40, 41, 50, 60, 61, 78, 83, 90, 91, 94, 107, 111, 113, 121, 127, 169
palm kernel oil, 57
pancreas, 18, 29, 48, 49
panic, 126, 160, 163
parasites, 15, 23, 28, 33, 57
Parkinson, 11, 111, 126, 127, 128, 129, 166
penis, 109, 133, 134
pepsin, 46
peptides, 95
Peroxidation, 82
pH, 24, 25, 26, 31, 35, 37, 39, 46, 53, 64, 65, 106, 123, 162, 163
phosphorus, 24, 37, 96
phytates, 49
phytochemicals, 4, 71, 77, 95
phytosterols, 95
Pine Bark, 87
pineal, 100, 118
pituitary, 74, 94, 98, 134, 160, 168
plant enzymes, 18, 46, 47, 53, 125
platelets, 108, 116
PMS, 26, 60, 66, 89, 160
postmenopausal, 113
potassium, 24, 62, 66, 71, 82, 114, 124
PREG, 99
premature aging, 14, 53, 82
premature ejaculation, 134
progesterone, 24, 75, 93, 94, 95, 96, 97, 99, 100, 109, 117, 122, 124, 125, 164, 167, 171, 183
Progesterone U.S.P., 95
Propolis, 72
prostaglandins, 58, 59, 132, 134
prostate, 71, 94, 100, 130, 131, 132, 164, 167, 168
protease, 46, 49, 125, 165, 169
protein, 17, 32, 37, 39, 41, 45, 46, 48, 49, 52, 62, 63, 64, 65, 67, 90, 91, 133, 167

protesin, 17, 32, 37, 39, 41, 45, 46, 48, 49, 52, 62, 63, 64, 65, 67, 68, 69, 70, 71, 89, 90, 91, 106, 111, 128, 133, 162, 163, 166, 167
psyllium, 28
rheumatoid arthritis, 52, 104, 144
Rhodeola rosea, 127
ringing of the ears, 59
RNA/DNA, 67
royal jelly, 27, 72, 100, 103, 105, 123, 125, 168

S-T

S.O.D., 50, 84
SAC, 84
saliva, 17, 18, 93
Sarsaparilla, 97
Saw Palmetto, 132, 133
sea vegetables, 40, 65, 69, 92, 136, 161, 168
selenium, 36, 51, 63, 82
semen, 130
vitamin D, 37, 124
vitamins, 7, 8, 17, 18, 19, 21, 26, 27, 31, 32, 37, 39, 46, 50, 58, 61, 62, 63, 66, 68, 69, 72, 82, 96, 112, 129, 157, 158, 159, 160, 162, 164, 165, 166, 168, 183
vomiting, 25
waste, 17, 19, 20, 21, 28, 29, 38, 58, 103, 104, 114, 131, 159
water retention, 92, 94, 98
wheat grass, 61, 62, 63, 68, 169
wheatgrass, 64, 123, 138
white blood cells, 47, 141
wild yam, 95, 96, 99, 117, 118, 164, 183
worms, 28
wrinkle, 1, 53, 59, 89, 91
wrinkles, 4, 30, 45, 51, 59, 74, 75, 89, 160
yeast, 19, 32, 33, 36, 48, 76, 105, 163, 164, 169, 183
zinc, 36, 41, 42, 49, 50, 56, 58, 63, 82, 96, 108, 124, 130, 132, 167